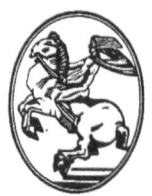

ACTA NEUROCHIRURGICA
SUPPLEMENTUM 27

Ludwig M. Auer

The Pathogenesis of Hypertensive Encephalopathy

**Experimental Data
and Their Clinical Relevance
With Special Reference
to Neurosurgical Patients**

SPRINGER-VERLAG
WIEN NEW YORK

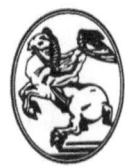

Ludwig Michael Auer, M.D.
Neurosurgical Department (Head: Prof. Dr. F. Heppner),
University of Graz, Graz, Austria

With 46 partly colored Figures

Library of Congress Cataloging in Publication Data. Auer, Ludwig M. 1948–   . The pathogenesis of hypertensive encephalopathy. (Acta neurochirurgica: Supplementum; 27.) 1. Cerebrovascular disease. 2. Hypertension — Complications and sequelae. 3. Brain damage. 4. Diseases — Animal models. I. Title. II. Series. RC388.5A93. 616.8'1. 78-15534.

ISBN-13:978-3-211-81490-1   e-ISBN-13:978-3-7091-8522-3
DOI: 10.1007/978-3-7091-8522-3

To Eva Verena

Preface

This monograph aims to provide a survey of recent research on the pathogenesis of hypertensive encephalopathy. Or, in other words, to relate experimental results directly to a clinical problem. I am convinced that a very important task of experimental medical research is to find applications to the relevant clinical problem as soon as possible, and to avoid distraction by an increasingly overwhelming accumulation of new information from all fields of scientific work. This is undoubtedly easier for a clinician than for a scientist who is only concerned with fundamental research; successful research for clinical medicine thus requires that clinicians and scientific specialists in the theoretical medical branches cooperate with each other. To fulfill this aim the clinician must be able to think in pathophysiological terms to a considerable extent, which will scarcely be possible if he is involved in routine clinical medicine alone.

Experimental work thus presents a real challenge to the physician who wishes to solve a medical problem and also possesses scientific curiosity. Besides an answer to his question, he has the opportunity to obtain a real feeling for what he has learned to call "physiological". I hope with my own experimental work to provide a convincing example of how such work may serve as an impressive reminder to the clinician of the possibly grave consequences of underestimating a development in the course of a serious illness, for instance a hypertensive episode following head injury.

Regarding the experimental facilities available to me, I am above all indebted to my teacher, the head of the Neurosurgical Clinic in Graz, Professor F. Heppner, whose efforts made our brain-research laboratory reality, for his continuous and generous support of my work. The considerable financial support provided by the "Österreichischer Fonds zur Förderung der wissenschaftlichen Forschung" covered most of the instrumentation for the laboratory.

I should also like to express my gratitude to Barbro Johansson and Eric T. MacKenzie for their critical contributions to this text.

Graz, June 1978   Ludwig M. Auer

Contents

1. Introduction

Prior to the work of Oppenheimer and Fishburg in 1928 [222], it was generally assumed that cerebral symptoms during hypertension were derived from uremia that was caused by renal failure. The authors stated that the cerebral symptoms were independent of renal insufficiency and called the clinical picture "hypertensive encephalopathy". This syndrome is known to be present with a number of neurological deficits such as paresis or paresthesia and visual disturbances and leading to generalized convulsions and coma. Starting with dizziness and headache, hypertensive encephalopathy can end in a lethal outcome.

Hypertensive crises are not only just an observation combined with clinical symptoms in different fields of medicine but also a source of such complications as intracranial hematomata and brain edema. In a recent study, about 75% of patients (200 in total) with cerebral infarction were found to suffer from fixed or fluctuating hypertension [53]. Seventy-one percent of 224 patients with non-traumatic intracerebral hematomata were hypertensive [189]. It was, therefore, a challenge for experimental medicine to determine the pathophysiological and morphological background to hypertensive encephalopathy and associated brain edema. F. B. Byrom was one of the first to study extensively the cerebrovascular changes in animals made hypertensive by stenosing a renal artery after contralateral nephrectomy. He began his work between 1930 and 1940. In his 1954 publication [55] he described cerebrovascular changes in hypertensive rats in which he found that increasing arterial pressure *per se* did not yet provoke hypertensive encephalopathy in the sense of clinical signs. Only when the already hypertensive rat suffered an additional rise in pressure did Byrom observe such clinical symptoms as seizures, weakness, apathy and coma. These same animals had brain edema, alterations of pial vessel diameters and sometimes morphological changes in the arterial vessel walls. Similar observations could be made on normal kidney in the hypertensive rats, but they were not seen in the kidney that was protected against hypertension by the clip which stenosed the renal artery. Thus it became apparent that the increase in arterial pressure caused the observed changes, and that hypertensive encephalopathy was a cerebrovascular disease. Now, pial vessel changes to various stimuli had been observed as early as 1928, when Forbes [106] and 10 years later Fog [101, 102] presented their results with the window technique. Those were the first experimental data giving evidence that there is an active regulation of cerebral vessels and not just passive pressure-dependent diameter changes [242]. It could be inferred from their data that the contrary of pressure-passive behavior is the case: namely, constriction with increasing, and dilatation with decreasing arterial pressure. Although Forbes and Fog had observed some instances of pial vasodilatation during acute hypertension, Byrom thought vaso-constriction to be the more probable pathological event. Byrom considered vasodilatation and subsequent high filtration pressure, but somewhat misleading results of carotid flow measurements during hypertension led him to the opinion that the Bayliss effect [30] acted on vessels with high intraluminal pressure, and that this effect could lead to excessive vasoconstriction and later on to ischemic edema.

Byrom's observations of pial vessels were performed without taking control micrographs from the normal vessels at normal CO_2 tension. Therefore, it was not really possible to judge what was a normal diameter and what was spasm or dilatation, assuming that there were not enormous changes in vessel diameter. Similar results were obtained by Rodda and Denny-Brown [237, 238] using the chronic renal hyper-tension model in monkeys: 1 to 19 weeks after partially occluding both renal arteries, they observed pial vessels by means of an open cranial-window technique. They described changes in arteriolar dia-meters with alternate, segmental constriction and dilatation and called their observation the "sausage-string effect" or "cork-screws". Constrictions between dilated segments were described as being so excessive as to make the vessel nearly invisible and to produce stasis. In histological sections, they saw early stage arteriolonecrosis in areas in which there were vessel diameter changes and Trypan-blue exu-dations.

These two experimental series of Byrom and Rodda/Denny-Brown are somewhat different from those performed by Meyer et al. in 1960 [209], who had observed diffuse pial arteriolar constriction in a more acute stage of renal and drug-induced hypertension, and Molnar [211], who observed a decrease in cerebral blood flow in rabbits during acute hypertension induced by electrical stimulation of the brain stem. But all of these experiments have one conclusion in common: the assumption that focal arteriolar overconstriction indicates that there can be areas of preserved or exaggerated autoregulation, where, later on, arteriolonecrosis might occur during experimental hypertension.

These studies brought about a great impetus for further experimental work. The main interest of later, acute experiments was to discover the pathogenesis of encephalopathy. I myself felt that the most relevant question was: is it really vasospasm or is it vasodilatation that leads to cerebral dysfunction? And, does brain edema occur during or after an acute arterial pressure increase?

Early results, of great interest and consequence, were obtained from another vascular bed and were published by Giese [120]. Intestinal arteries, observed during angiotensin-induced acute hypertension in rats, exhibited segmentally shaped diameter changes with constricted and dilated portions. Three hours later, colloidal carbon particles were present in the arteriolar wall of dilated segments only, and never in constricted segments. This, the first argument for vasodilatation to be the basis for hypertensive encephalopathy, received further support from blood flow measurements that indicated increased flow during acute hypertension [83]. Lassen and Agnoli [187] called the upper limit of cerebrovascular autoregulation, beyond which there was a pressure-passive increase in cerebral blood flow, "breakthrough of cerebral autoregulation by excessive hypertension". To test this hypothesis, a number of experiment series have been performed which deserve summary.

The term "hypertensive encephalopathy" lacks a clearcut definition and is commonly used for the neurological dysfunction seen during acute arterial hypertension both in previously hypertensive and in previously normotensive subjects. The two situations, however, namely acute hypertension in previously normotensive and previously hypertensive individuals may well not be the same. In the context of an acute arterial pressure increase in the chronic situation, I should like to recall Byrom's chronically hypertensive rats which had clinical symptoms when, and only when, an additional steep rise in pressure occurred. Some of the observed changes were very similar to recent results in experiments with acutely induced hypertension, but a significant difference might be found in animal studies after periods of hypertension longer than 5 minutes or so. Furthermore, the histological picture of vessel-wall changes after repeated acute, or chronically high blood pressures might differ also, as will be discussed in later chapters.

It was the use of different methods by different investigators that led to the assumption that high blood pressure was the originating factor of encephalopathy. Renal hypertension, blood-pressure increases induced by clamping of the thoracic aorta and drug-induced hypertension were all followed by patchy cortical extravasations. High intraluminal pressure thus became the most probable cause of these changes. But it could not be just the fact of high pressure alone, because Byrom [55] had observed a great number of chronically hypertensive rats with blood pressure around or above 200 mm Hg without clinical symptoms of hypertensive encephalopathy and morphological signs of cerebrovascular changes, except when an additional hypertensive crisis added to the already existent hypertension. Therefore, there had to be an acute onset of high intraluminal pressure to produce extravasation and this was in fact proven by Häggendal and Johansson, who increased carotid intraluminal pressure selectively [124] and performed experiments [125] in two series of cats, in which blood pressure was elevated abruptly in one series and stepwise in the other. Stepwise increase failed to elicit extravasation, whereas a number of the animals in the acute pressure increase group showed the typical cortical Evans-blue extravasation. But what protected the other acutely hypertensive animals from cortical extravasation? At this point I wanted to test the hypothesis that the steepness and/or percentage degree of blood-pressure increase is responsible for cerebrovascular alteration and formation of edema. Therefore, my own work has dealt with neuropathological findings in previously healthy and normotensive cats; findings were obtained during or immediately after an acute increase in arterial pressure. In my own experiments, performed at nearly the same time as those of the Glasgow group [196, 89], I examined vascular reactivity while avoiding any harm to the pial surface during opening of the skull and using a closed-window technique.

In a further approach, I was interested especially in the localization of early extravasation. Here, attention was focused on lesions in the arteriolar wall described by Giese [120] and Johansson, who observed Evans-blue extravasations around arterioles in fluorescence-microscopic preparations. In electron-microscopic studies, all types of vessels have been shown to be involved in BBB alteration during acute hypertension, but it is primarily arterioles that have been implicated. It appeared improbable to me that extravasation should take place only through dilated arterioles and not through capillaries. I therefore planned a study that involved intravital microangiography to see the very first sites of extravasation. Last, and by no means least, the number of studies performed in recent years seemed worth summarizing so as to clarify the important factors in the origin of hypertensive encephalopathy.

2. Methods

2.1. The Cranial Window Technique

2.1.1. Introduction and Historical Survey

2.1.1.1. Development of Technique

The first intravital microscopic observations were reported by Leeuwenhoek, the inventor of the microscope. Examination of the brain surface dates back to the 19th Century, in the publications of Ravina (1811) and Donders (1850) [72]. The first systematic intravital-microscopic investigations were begun in the second decade of our century. In 1925, Heimberger [133] studied the capillary bed in human skin with a simple microscope and carbon light source and gave the first important report on capillary reactions to localized trauma. Landis [182] and Forbes [107], using similar instruments, first observed and described frog mesentery using a "Photomikroskopisches Okular" from Zeiss. Wolff and Fog used normal microscopes without adaptation, as phototechnical possibilities were very restricted. Quantitative evaluation had to be performed by directly observing the object because suitable light sources for photo-documentation at higher magnifications did not exist. The "bright-field-opaque-illuminator" optic, described in 1923 by Vonwiller [280] was not able to improve conditions for intravital, direct-light microscopy and this system was rarely used. In 1932, Heine [134] with his dark-ground-illuminator created the basis of the modern "ultropak" system. The next important step was probably the development of a high-pressure mercury lamp (Gottschewski [121]). This lamp made fluorescence angiography possible with photometrical and movie documentation; the method of fluorescence microangiography by itself was a great advancement (Teichmann [276]). In 1955, Peters [226] gave a very extensive survey of the intravital microscopic technique, mentioning the problems and, especially, the sources of error that were due to surgical procedures. For the first time, a photometrical stand with vibration-absorber fitting and a gliding object table were used. At the same time Zweifach was using an intravital microscope device for his studies on microcirculation [293] which were based upon excellent methodological studies [294]. In 1958, Gemählich [116] summarized the advantages of the "ultropak" illuminator.

The investigation of capillary function is generally coupled with the name of L. Illig. In 1961, he presented an extensive survey on the microcirculation as seen by microscopy [148]. Extensive work on the technology of intravital microscopy has been done since by Brånemark [38, 39, 45—49]. Other advances in this field were achieved by the image-splitting technique which allows *in-vivo* measurements of pial vessels [28, 73], and the use of video systems which permit many technical advances such as the measurement of flow velocity and vessel diameters [27, 149, 150, 212].

Whereas nearly everybody presently studying the pial vasculature uses the direct-light darkfield optic system with a cool light, xenon, Hg-pressure lamp or flash-light source, the surgical techniques for the preparation of the cortical surface, which have always differed in the past, still differ.

2.1.1.2. The Brain Surface

"I think not least is the real fun of working at it. You never know what will turn up next. It is like exploring an unclimbed mountain."
H. S. Forbes

The most fascinating of all scientific work is perhaps the direct observation of a biological phenomenon because we are immediately confronted with changes. We are, at a glance, able to see the effects of a drug and natural events without the aid of mathematics or other indirect techniques. In this sense the words of Forbes, quoted above, should be interpreted in the light of my own experience on the subject, fascinated as I am myself.

So much the more impressive must have been the first views of the exposed brain surface of a living being as, at the beginning of scientific medicine and biology this organ was practically taboo. After the first systematic observation of pial vessels by Florey [98], this branch of brain research has been mainly connected with the name of Henry S. Forbes [107—112], together with Wolff [289, 290] and some others [94, 95, 229, 261]—these workers presenting the first important results on cerebral blood flow and its regulation. Forbes' technique, imitated and modified by a great number of investigators, consists chiefly of replacing the parietal skull bone with a lucite window fixed tightly into a metal frame. Care taken during craniotomy and the avoidance of any pressure on the cortical area after opening of the dura should allow observation of reactive pial vessels which are bathed with warm cerebrospinal fluid.

Finesinger [94, 95], Pool [229], Fog [100—103], Beickert [34], Chorobski and Penfield [57] used this method and so initiated the first fundamental discussions on the regulatory mechanisms of the cerebral circulation.

In 1938, Clark [58] assessed a cranial window, modified from one by Wentsler for the rabbit ear, used without anesthesia for periods of 4 months or more. But the advantage of a relatively physiological situation had to be balanced against two disadvantages which very soon put an end to this procedure: firstly, animals never kept quiet enough to allow observations under high magnifications; and secondly, a thin membrane developed between cranial window and brain surface—sometimes after some days, sometimes only after weeks, making further investigations impossible by veiling the vessels.

The investigations by the group of Clark and Forbes were followed by the publications of Villaret [279] who used a similar method; his "bull's eye" (French: "hublot") could remain in place for weeks, but led to the same problems as those of Wentsler's technique.

In 1944, Shelden and Pudenz [258] published experimental results where the whole calvarium was replaced by an artificial one, inserted over several surgical sessions. Minard [210] reevaluated this method and reported decisive disadvantages and impediments that included infection by CSF leakage. The time taken for the operation (in four sessions) and the intensive care of the animals (over weeks) made him drop this as a viable procedure.

The original method of Forbes, on the other hand, is still used for investigations into the cerebral circulation. It is carried out both with a window [236] and without replacement of the cranial bone defect [2, 240, 241, 245—250, 281, 283].

It was in 1955 or so that experimental intravital microscopy was begun in our clinic by F. Heppner [135—137] and J. E. Marx who used an incident-light microscope (Reichert, Vienna) and an open cranial-window technique.

2.1.2. Description of the Present Method

2.1.2.1. Operative Procedure

As experimental animals, 50 cats of either sex—weighing between 1.5 and 3.5 kg—were used. The cats were anesthetized with 35 mg/kg Nembutal, intubated endotracheally and respirated with a $4:1$ mixture of $N_2O : O_2$, using a Loosco respirator. One femoral vein and artery were cannulated for medication, continuous arterial pressure monitoring and frequent withdrawal of arterial samples to estimate pH, P_aCO_2 and P_aO_2. Arterial pressure is continuously measured directly via the femoral catheter and a Statham P 23 dB transducer linked to a Rikadenki-cassette writer. Blood gases and pH are monitored with an AVL Gas Check. The present cranial window corresponds to the methods of Forbes [116], Schmidt [245] and Heppner [135]. The window is made in the right parietal region; after opening the skin by a sagittal incision, periosteum and temporal muscle are drawn aside. During irrigation of the calvarium with 37 °C Ringer's solution, the bone is removed with a dental drill or a hand-driven trephan, until a very thin bone membrane remains over the dura, thus preventing direct trauma to dura and brain by the drill head. This thin layer of bone is hooked with a fine needle and removed with fine dissecting forceps, so leaving a ring of 1–2 mm on the periphery as a support for the glass window.

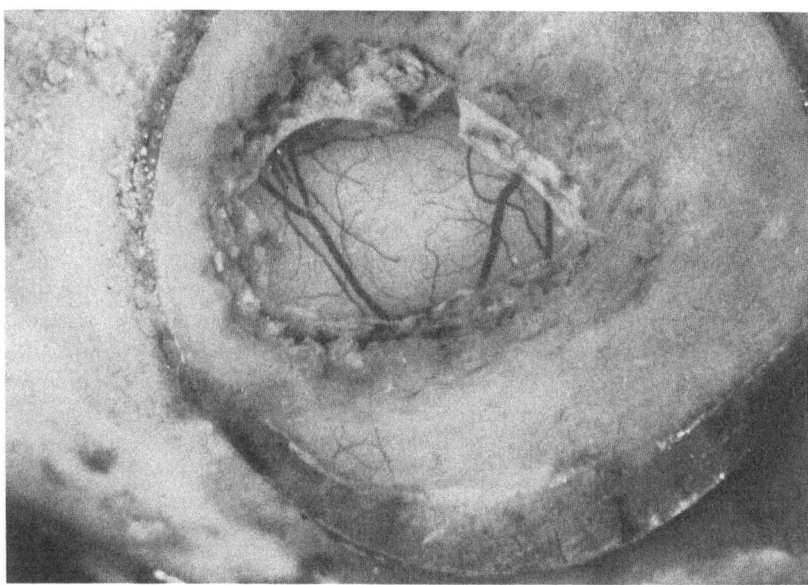

Fig. 1. Parietal glass window in a cat, sealed with acrylic, reveals a single gyrus

A similar procedure is performed with the dura, where greater vessels are co-agulated with bipolar microforceps. In the end the pial surface is visible over an area of about 100 mm². The dura is opened under microscopy using 40-fold magnification. Finally, a glass window on a metal frame, similar to that of Forbes or a glass window without metal frame, is placed over the craniotomy and fixed with either acrylic or dental cement (Fig. 1). Accordingly, cerebrospinal fluid is prevented from escaping and a more or less physiological situation is reestablished within the intracranial compartments. Two holes in the metal frame with small needles affixed allow remove of air bubbles and administration of pharmacological substances to the cortical surface and the pial vessels.

2.1.2.2. Technical Equipment

The basic instrument was a "Leitz-Intravitalmikroskop" (Figs. 2 a, b). Besides a heavy arm for objectives and illumination boxes, it possesses a column for fixation of either a movie or a still camera, both mounted on a vibration-damped table. The microscope stage consists of an animal fixation table in a sort of tub,

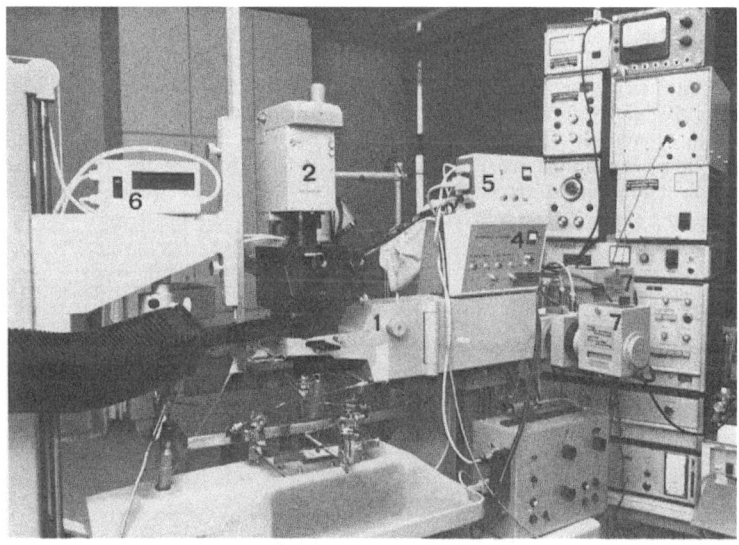

Fig. 2 a. Leitz "Intravitalmikroskop" and physiological control unit. *1* three-way tube for observation, photography and photometry; *2* still camera; *3* Ultropak objective; *4* control unit for electronic slips; *5* electronic timer for measurement of experiment duration; *6* digital display of mean arterial blood pressure; *7* light sources

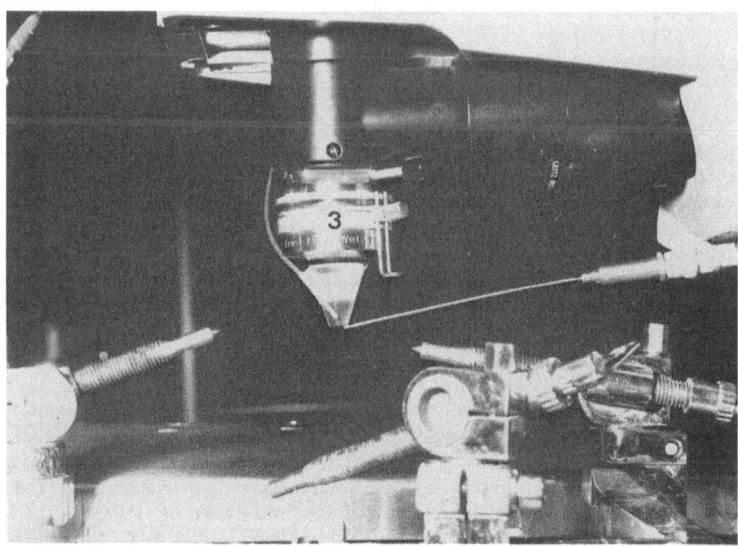

Fig. 2 b. Ultropak objective with temperature sensor and irrigation tube

freely movable by micro- or macrotransmission. Light sources are a 60 W low-voltage lamp, a Xenon lamp and a high-pressure Hg lamp (200 W/4, Leitz, Wetzlar). For incident light microscopy, the "ultropak" is a good objective system, sufficient for movie and photographical documentation. Magnifications between 40- and 400-fold were used. The "ultropak" is a dark-field system with pancratic condenser (Fig. 2 c). Especially with the immersion cap, the plane object side of which is separated from the cortical window by a thin film of irrigation fluid, the "ultropak" allows careful work. For special fluorescence-

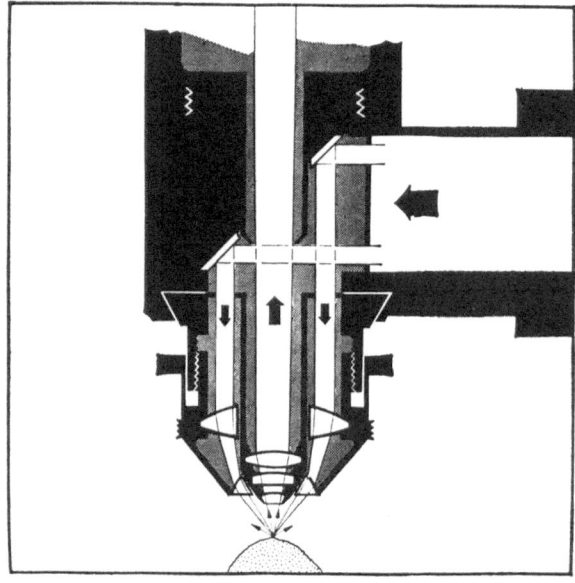

Fig. 2 c. Function of Ultropak objective with ring condensor

angiographic observations, a "ploem-opak" system was used, equipped with filter combinations to produce excitation light in a specified range of wave lengths. The surface temperature of the cranial glass window is controlled with a DISA type 14905 thermosensor. The surface is held constant at 37 °C by irrigating the outer surface of the glass window with fluid (saline, Ringer's solution), which is thermostatically controlled (Thermomix, Braun-Melsungen). The procedure of irrigating the window surface is necessary, since all the light sources used give off heat, although all of them have a special heat-protection filter in their housing. To investigate temperature changes produced by single light sources and filter combinations, heat production was measured at a distance of 1 mm from the objective surface and is given in Table 1. It shows different values of temperature increase with different filters. With filter combinations used commonly for direct observation, temperature remains unchanged within a range of + 01. °C for low-voltage illumination, of 0.3 °C for the Xenon lamp and 0.8 °C for the high-pressure Hg lamp. During photography or cinematography, it is not possible to use all these filters because the exposure times would become too

Table 1. *Temperature Changes Caused by Different Light Sources, Measured at a Distance of 1 mm From Objective Immersion Cap*

Light source	Room temperature	Temperature directly under the objective	Reduced to room temperature by following filters
Wolfram LV-lamp	23 °C	24.1 °C	0.2% grey filter (NG 3)
Xenon	23 °C	32.5 °C	5% grey filter (NG 4), green filter
Hg	23 °C	> 40 °C	2 mm BG 12 CS 3-73 (λ 410 mμ) Kalflex heat filter

Table 2. *Temperature Changes With Different Light Sources, Measured at a Distance of 1 mm From the Objective Immersion Cap in the Irrigation Fluid on the Cranial Window*

Light source	Brain surface temperature with direct illumination, without irrigation	Normal brain surface temperature by following irrigation procedure
Wolfram LV-lamp	37.6 °C	200 ml/hour 37 °C
Xenon-lamp	46 °C	250 ml/hour 37 °C
Hg-lamp + 2 mm BG 12 CS 3-73, Kalflex	37.8 °C	250 ml/hour 37 °C

long. Therefore, at such times the irrigation system is switched to a higher flow level than during simple observation. The attempt at optimal heat protection was improved further with an electronic slip device which opened just for the time of exposure during the use of high-intensity light. Such slips are placed on the outlet of each light source, one serving for direct observation and one for photographic documentation. It is linked to an automatic timer that acts precisely during film exposure and closes the observation light source and opens the strong Xenon light source during exposure time [15]. The photographic equipment itself consists of a Leitz "Orthomat" camera with electronic exposure timing. Movies (16 mm) are made with a Bolex camera. For black and white pictures, Ilford Pan F, HP 4, FP 4 and Kodak Proceeding are used. Color pictures were taken with "Kodachrome high speed EHB 135" and „Agfachrome 50 L". For 16 mm movie films, "Ektachrome 7242" and "Kodak Eastman 4-X 7224" were chosen. The development of black and white pictures is made at 800–1,000 ASA and of color pictures at 800 ASA. Movie films are developed in a special laboratory. Single measurements of pial vessel diameter were made from magnified slides. For determination of absolute size, a micrometer scale (Leitz,

Wetzlar) was photographed and projected with the same optical systems as the photographs. In the control experiments, repeated diameter measurements under steady-state conditions led to a mean diameter fluctuation of $\pm$ 0.83%.

For continuous monitoring of vessel diameter changes, a photomultiplyer (Knott-Elektronik, Munich) was placed into the ocular raypath instead of the still or movie camera [16]. Power (8.5 kV) was produced by a Knott high-stability power supply, type NSHM, BN 600. The object was illuminated with a 12 V lamp which was stabilized with a Leitz power stabilizer. Light intensity changes were documented continuously on a Rikadenki 2-channel writer, model TCO 2010. A Leitz S 525 "Selektions-Interferenz-Filter" was used to eliminate all wave-lengths except green and to send a green and black picture into the photomultiplier. Thus, the bright color of the brain surface appeared green; vessels, however, were black and the photomultiplier continuously measured the intensity of green light. The intensity is decreased when more vessels are present and increased the fewer there are. The same also occurs when single vessels dilate or constrict; when a pial vessel dilates, the black compartment becomes larger, and *vice versa*. At low magnification, many vessels are in the objective field and the intensity represents an overall mean picture of vascular reactivity. At higher magnification, single vessels down to 20–30 μm can be observed under 300–400-fold magnification.

The relationship between changes of intensity and percentage changes in vascular diameter is unknown. The method gives, nevertheless, a very precise impression of the time course of vessel reactions to various stimuli. The method thus presents a useful way to study the dynamics of pial vessel diameter. Slight, rhythmical changes of pial vessel diameter become measurable (see also chapter "Results"). Reactions shown on the intensity reading can be verified by direct observation. Using the surface of a cat cadaver brain as a control, the photometric output is a straight line without any upward or downward deflection.

2.1.3. Performance of Experiments

2.1.3.1. CO$_2$-Reactivity Test

At the beginning of each experiment, cerebrovascular responsiveness was tested by inducing hyper- and hypocapnia. The cats were ventilated with 5–10% CO$_2$ added to the respiratory gas mixture. After a hypercapnic period of less than a minute (check by blood-gas analysis), a period of hyperventilation followed, until a hypocapnic P$_a$CO$_2$ was established. During hypocapnia, MABP remained more or less constant (mean 102 mm Hg) except in one cat, where MABP decreased from 110 to 60 mm Hg. During hypercapnia, increases in MABP of 10–20 mm Hg were often seen. Photographs were taken before, during and after changes in P$_a$CO$_2$.

Single results are given in Table 3. The changes in P$_a$O$_2$ were followed by characteristic diameter changes in all cats—*i.e.* dilatation during hypercapnia in all vessels and constriction during hypocapnia in arterial vessels (Figs. 3 to 5) [23, 231]. Dilatation was much more evident in arterial than venous vessels. Small vessels showed higher percentage changes than larger ones (Fig. 4). An individual example is given in Figs. 5 a–c which shows pial vessels at different levels of P$_a$CO$_2$.

During hypercapnia P$_a$CO$_2$ was increased from 35–43.5 mm Hg (mean 37.9 mm Hg) to 47–117 mm Hg (mean 67.2 mm Hg). Arterial vessels with a resting diameter of more than 30 μm (37–120 μm, mean 57 μm) dilated to + 34.7% over resting values, *i.e.* to 32.1–176.3 μm (mean 83.2 μm) (see Fig. 3). Arterial

Table 3

Exp.	PₐCO₂	Vessel diameters in μm										
F 59	36	65	55	45	27.5	35						
	20	57.5	50	42.5	27.5	30						
F 56	23	27.5	22.5	32.5	30	40						
	68	40	42.5	50	60	55						
F 53	45	90	90	15	17.5	87.5	87.5	15		12.5	67.5	
	95	95	110	35	30	100	110	20		20	80	
F 52	39	35		17.5	17.5	7.5						
	73	42.5		25	27.5	17.5						
F 51	36	47.5	55	25	45	35	30	55				
	17	50	42.5	12.5	35	20	22.5	45				
F 48	42	67.5	50	37.5	35	55	35	12.5	10			
	33	57.5	45	35	30	60	32.5	15	7.5			
F 46	36	37.5	30	27.5	15							
	47	42.5	37.5	35	17.5							
F 41	42	46.2	48.4	64.5	63							
	49	52.4	50.2	64.5	71							
F 38	44	176.3	167.7	167.7	163.4	21.5	34.4					
	60	206.4	215	210.7	206.4	38.7	43					
F 37	39	46.2	49.3	53.9	33.9	30.8	30.8					
	56	50.8	53.9	61.6	35.4	35.4	35.4					
F 27	38	54.6	41.6	23.4	13	7.8						
	69	57.2	57	33.8	23.4	10.4						
	16	41.6	37.7	18.2	17.6	7.8						
F 61	38	40	40	30	30	22.5	15	15	15	40	35	
	47	70	65	60	50	35	32.5	20	22.5	80	65	
F 61	38	20	15									
	47	35	25									
F 64	30	10	95	90	95							
	84	35	185	140	140							
F 64	30	30	30	30	30	20	20	25	20	20	15	
	84	40	42.5	37.5	35	35	20	52.5	37.5	42.5	30	
F 65	41	85	80	60	55	50	40					
	102	100	100	80	80	80	55					
	30	65	67.5	57.5	52.5	50	40					
F 69	41	35	40	45	50	20	40	45	20	30		
	124	45	55	60	65	30	50	55	60	30	50	
	25	30	30	35	35	15			50			
F 71	36	30	55	55	55	55	20					
	52	55	75	75	60	60	20					
F 72 I	38	15	15	15	40	42.5	47.5	40	50	5	5	5
	100	30	30	30	70	75	80	75	75	30	25	20
F 72 II	28	130	115	120	15	12.5	15	15	25	15	10	5
	67	170	160	165	25	15	30	35	30	30	27.5	10

vessels up to 30 μm (5–30 μm, mean 18 μm) showed a diameter increase of 92.8%, *i.e.* to 17.5–42.5 μm (mean 31.9 μm), nearly a threefold dilatation when compared to arterioles over 30 μm in resting diameter.

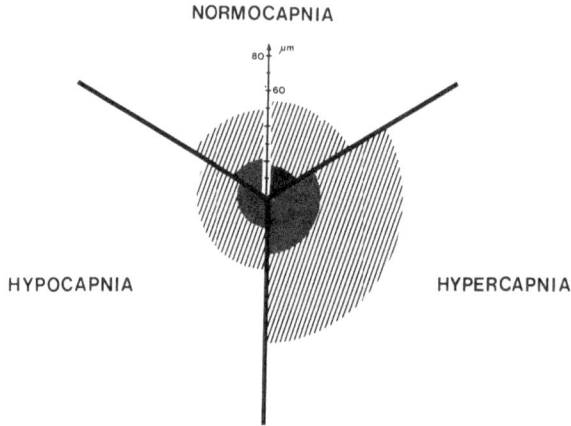

Fig. 3. Mean arterial diameter changes in μm after transition from normocapnia to
hypo- or hypercapnia. Inner circles: vessels with initial diameter ≤ 30 μm; outer
circles: vessels > 30 μm

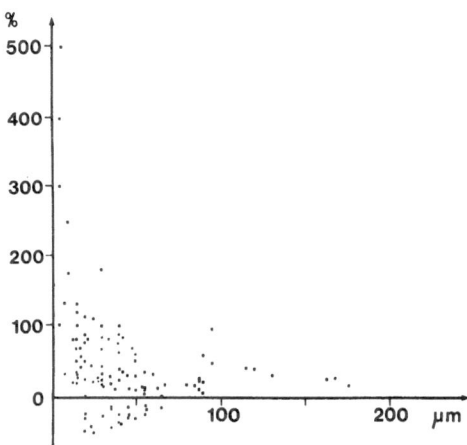

Fig. 4. Resting diameters of pial arterial vessels in μm plotted against percentage
changes during hypercapnia and hypocapnia. The curvilinear relationship can be
seen, with greater dilatation of the smaller vessels than of the larger ones

During hypocapnia P_aCO_2 was lowered from 35–45 mm Hg to 17–33 mm Hg
(mean 24.6 mm Hg). Arterial constriction in vessels over 30 μm was — 13.9 on
average, i.e. from 35–85 μm (mean 50.2 μm) to 20–67.5 μm (mean 42.6 μm)
(see Fig. 3). Arteriolar vessels under 30 μm (10–30 μm, mean 21.7 μm) constricted
to 7.5–27.5 μm (mean 17.6 μm) for a percentage decrease of 16.9%.

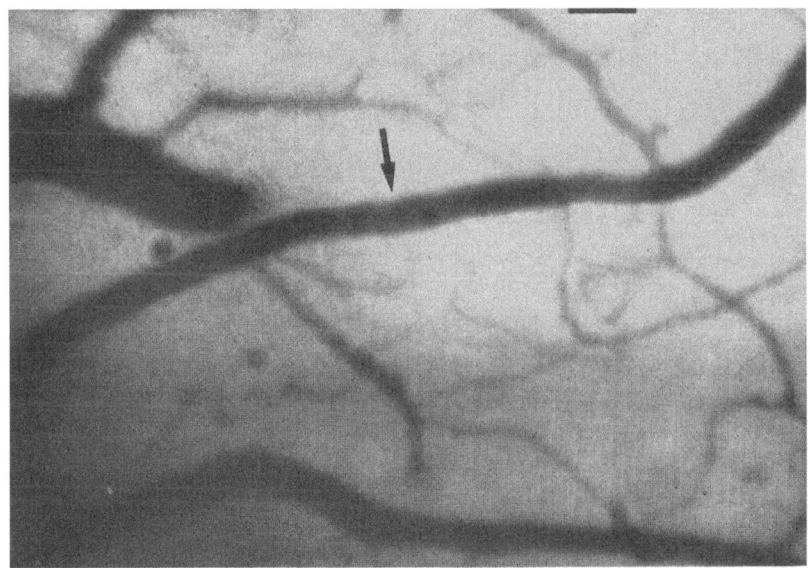

Fig. 5 a

Fig. 5. Pial vascular conditions at different levels of arterial CO_2 tension and constant MABP. Black line = 113 μm, arrow indicates arteriole. a) P_aCO_2 = 38 mm Hg; b) P_aCO_2 = 67 mm Hg; c) P_aCO_2 = 16 mm Hg

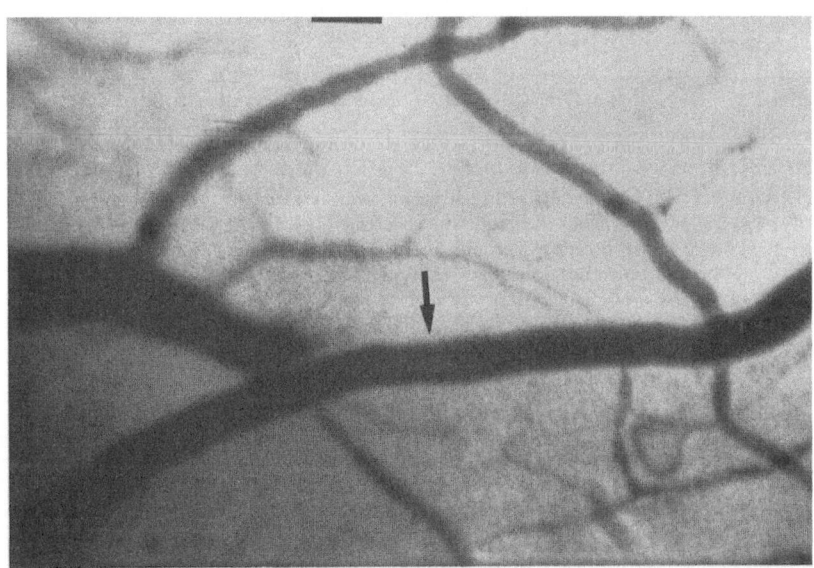

Fig. 5 b

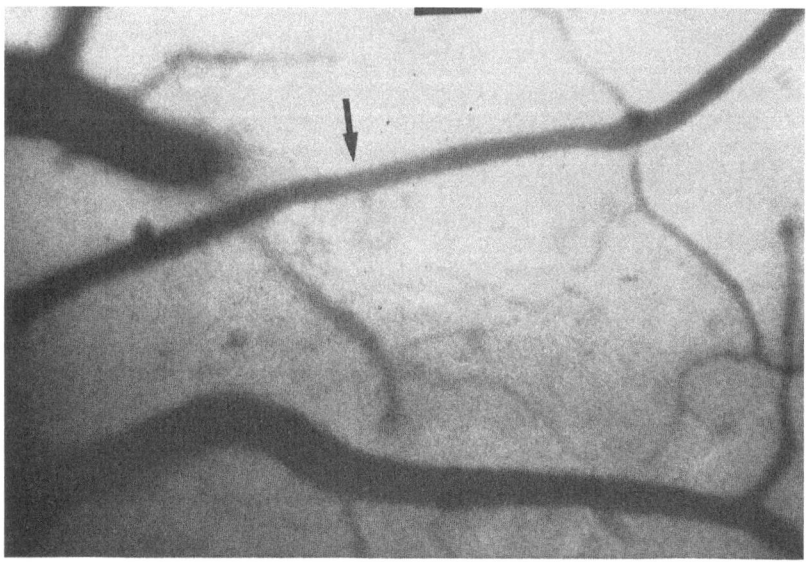

Fig. 5 c

In six cats the onset of vasodilatation during hypercapnia was examined with photometric techniques (Fig. 11). Vasodilatation occurred within 7–48 seconds (mean 19 seconds). Further data, however, would go beyond the scope of this work and are described in detail in a separate paper [23].

2.1.3.2. Induction of Acute Hypertension

The experiments on pial vessel reactions during acutely induced hypertension were performed in three groups of cats, 39 in all.

Group 1: In 17 cats, acute hypertension was induced by intravenous injection of 10 µg/kg Hypertensin® (angiotensin-II-amide) (54,235). Angiotensin is known to increase arterial pressure without increasing cardiac output by increasing the total peripheral resistance, although individual organ resistances vary widely [201]. In 10 cats the experiment was performed at normal pH and normocapnia. Three experiments were performed under hypocapnia, two under hypercapnia and acidosis, and one in alkalosis (see Table 4).

Group 2: In ten cats subsequent to the same procedure as in group 1, acute hypertension was induced by the intravenous administration of 5 µg/kg nor-epinephrine. In two cats of this group, metabolic alkalosis was induced by the intravenous administration of Na_2CO_3 solution. Six cats, pretreated as group 1 and 2, served as controls without hypertension.

Group 3: Six further cats were used to study the time course of vascular reactivity to acute hypertension more precisely. They were treated as group 2, but without the parallel injection of Evans blue. The photometric measurement unit was adapted to the microscope instead of the photographic camera. The data from 23 hypertensive cats were used to obtain more information on the "sausage-string" phenomenon, especially the narrow segments between the dilated portions of vessels. The following calculations were made: the percentage arteriolar diameter decrease from experiments with preserved autoregulation (*i.e.* diffusely constricting vessels during hypertension) was compared with the degree of constriction of narrow segments between dilated portions from those experiments in which the sausage-string phenomenon occurred. The following hypothesis was tested: a number of investigators have reported that there is a constancy of blood flow up to a certain upper limit of cerebrovascular autoregulation; this constant blood flow runs parallel with constriction of the resistance vessels. Now, if the narrow segments in a situation of disturbed autoregulation were to constrict excessively (in comparison to the degree of diffuse constriction during hypertension and preserved autoregulation) then, but only then, could a decreased flow through such spastic vessels be presumed. If the contrary occurs, or if the extent of constriction were to be found to be equal in both situations, the assumption of arteriolar spasm caused by acute hypertension would have to give way to the concept of vascular distension and increased filtration pressure.

2.2. Macroscopy and Microangiography

For the visualization of protein extravasation during hypertension, 1 ml/kg of a 2% solution of Evans blue in saline was injected intravenously in 17 cats. For microangiography, the Evans blue was given at the moment when arterial pressure began to rise after the injection of angiotensin. The Evans blue was administered immediately before induction of hypertension in the other cats. This former procedure should—in addition—give a clearer picture of local conditions of flow phenomena during the first 20 seconds following the induction of hypertension, and an Evans-blue angiogram was made by taking a photograph every second for 15 seconds. Thereafter, a picture was taken at 20 and 30 seconds, and then every 30 seconds until 5 minutes after the initiation of hypertension. Furthermore, I especially wanted to examine the initial localization of extravasation and their relation to pial diameter changes during acute hypertension.

Six cats served as control and received only Evans blue. The Evans-blue angiograms were performed with the use of a variometer device (Wild-Heerbrugg). In six of the cats the cover glass was removed 5 minutes after the administration of angiotensin, the craniotomy was enlarged and the visible brain area photographed under a Zeiss surgical microscope within the subsequent 2 minutes.

2.3. Fluorescence Microscopy

For fluorescence microscopy, a series of 15 cats was investigated. They were treated in the same way as the other series, including intracranial pressure measurements [10]. In 10 cats, acute hypertension was produced by the intravenous injection of 10 µg/kg angiotensin. Five cats served as controls. Five minutes after beginning of hypertension and/or intravenous injection of 1 ml/kg 2% Evans blue, all cats were perfused with saline and 10% formaldehyde through an aortic cannula. After macroscopic inspection of Evans-blue extravasation, tissue samples were taken from cortex, white matter, basal ganglia and cerebellum for Evans-blue fluorescence microscopy. Thereafter, 10-µm thick frozen sections were cut in a Beckmann microtome, mounted on coverslips and viewed under a microscope, using a Hg lamp and a Schott UG 5 excitation filter.

2.4. Electron Microscopy

Preparations taken from cats of either sex were used for macroscopic and microscopic description of extravasation. Again, Evans blue was used to localize extravasated serum protein. Five minutes after the onset of hypertension, small pieces of cortical tissue were taken from areas stained blue, as well as from unstained areas. The tissues were put into 3% glutaraldehyde for 4 hours, thereafter into 1% osmium tetroxide buffered with cacodylate (pH 7.4). After dehydration in aethanolum, the tissues were embedded in Epon 812. Sections 20–40 nm thick were prepared on a Reichert Ultramikroton and observed in a Philips EM 200.

2.5. Measurement of Intracranial Pressure and Cerebral Venous Pressure

For estimation of cerebral perfusion pressure (CPP) which is the difference of systemic arterial pressure (SAP) and intracranial pressure (ICP), simultaneous SAP and ICP measurements were performed in a series of eight cats, anesthetized with sodium pentobarbital [11]. The cats were otherwise treated as in the experiments described above. Instead of the cranial window, a 1-mm PVC catheter was placed epidurally through a small burr hole and sealed with acrylic cement. Pressures were recorded using Statham P 23 dB transducers and the Hellige documentation unit. Hypertension was induced by the intravenous injection of angiotensin. Two cats served as controls. The extent of cortical protein extravasation was investigated using Evans blue as in the other experiments.

In a second series of five cats [25] anesthetized with 60 mg/kg alpha-chloralose and a 3 : 1 mixture of $N_2O : O_2$ and immobilized with 30 mg gallamine (Flaxedil®), simultaneous pressure recordings were made of arterial, cerebral venous and intracranial pressure. For these measurements a catheter was placed into the descending aorta via a femoral artery and another (Portex No. 2) into the superior sagittal sinus (SSS), 5–10 mm rostral to the torcular Herophili. The bone defect was covered with acrylic cement. A needle was placed percutaneously through the atlanto-occipital membrane into the cisterna magna for registration of CSF pressure changes. Femoral vein and artery were cannulated on one side. Thereafter, repeated acute hypertension was induced by the injection of 200 mg/kg metaraminol (Aramine®) at both normocapnic and hypercapnic levels of P_aCO_2. Finally, epileptic seizures were induced by intravenous injection of 1 mg/kg bicuculline which is known to cause maximal cerebral vasodilatation with a concomitant increase in arterial pressure [210, 166].

2.6. Discussion of Methods

2.6.1. The Window Technique

The window technique can be open to criticism and most careful control is necessary, since the operative procedures are rather extensive. Factors like direct trauma to pial vessels, excessive bleeding and changes in CSF composition might alter their reactivity to an undesirable extent. Microsurgical techniques are able to exclude vascular trauma. Hemorrhage can be avoided firstly by stopping bleeding out of the bony skull with bone wax before the last thin bone layer has been removed, secondly by careful bipolar coagulation of dural vessels. Homeostasis of CSF is achieved by sealing the window, thus surrounding the pial vessels with the animals' own CSF. The open-window technique is not recommended in longer physiological studies for several reasons. First of all, CSF homeostasis cannot be perfectly achieved. Secondly, the balance of intracranial compartments and thus of intracranial pressure and brain volume is altered, sooner or later leading to protrusion or even herniation of the brain [196].

Normal pial vessel reactivity could be shown by normal CO_2 reactivity [23]. Mistakes deriving from the measurement procedures are minimal, as shown with the control animals. Variations of diameter of about $\pm 1\%$ are negligible when compared to the changes measured during hypertension. These changes are, in addition, the same as reported by MacKenzie et al. [196] using an image-splitting eyepiece.

With all the qualification mentioned above, the intravital microscopic method is reliable for the observation of vascular reactions to different influences. It has become worthwhile due to technical innovation. Very careful manipulations and filtered light preserve normal arterial and venous relationships and allow their observation over a period of hours. Autoregulation remains, as has been reported by Forbes and Wolff [106], Fog [101], Forbes [110] and Schmidt [247].

The method does not apparently permit estimation of cerebral blood flow and its changes, as Sokoloff [262] wrote 18 years ago. Using the fluorescence-angiography technique in combination with the measurement of vessel diameter changes, the transit time of a fluorescent dye through the capillary bed can be a measure of blood flow changes. Furthermore, angiography is no longer restricted to measurements in "relatively large vessels" [262], but even permits investigation of the reaction of capillaries with diameters down to 5 μm. The greatest advantage of the angiographic method still seems to be the observation of diameter changes, although disturbances of the coagulatory system, evoked by the extrinsic or intrinsic factors can also be observed, as well as extravasation of dyes out of the vascular bed. Reports from Shelden and Pudenz [258], Minard [210], Schmidt [246] and Adler [2] indicate the value of intravital microscopy for the study of traumatized vessels.

2.6.2. The Photometric Measurements

The first results seem to indicate that photometrical evaluation of pial vessel diameter changes is an appropriate method for dynamic studies. In comparison to cinematographic and computer-assisted

TV methods [102, 103, 110, 111, 116, 133], it has the advantage of consisting of a simple device with direct and continuous documentation. The time course of reaction patterns can be studied easily. Besides the documentation of well-known pial arterial reactions to stimuli such as arterial pressure changes and hyper- or hypocapnia, the most interesting finding of this series of experiments was rhythmical diameter changes of such a slight degree that they could not be seen by simple microscopy. The proof for the assumption that grossly rising or falling of the photometric curve is due to vascular diameter changes, however, is the direct observation through the microscope. Rhythmical changes in cerebral tissue pO_2 have been reported by several authors but these pO_2 changes could not account for the observed changes in my series since the red light compartment was eliminated and rhythmical changes disappeared when measuring vessels at high magnifications, thus measuring the blood stream alone without surrounding brain tissue and without vessel walls [16].

2.6.3. Drugs Used for Production of Hypertension

Noradrenaline and angiotensin were used to elicit acute hypertension. Both were used not only to produce different blood-pressure patterns, but also so as not to base the whole investigation on a single agent and thereby to minimize interferences due to local effects. Noradrenaline, locally applied to the pial vessels, is known to cause constriction of pial arterial vessels, mainly those larger than 50 μm [113, 216, 282, 102, 106, 107, 234]. With regard to its effect on CBF, norepinephrine is known not to lower CBF [130, 134, 204] or to decrease CBF only to a minimal extent in both human [197] and animal experiments [264, 69, 235, 218]. These findings are similar to those obtained by sympathetic nerve stimulation [5, 67, 117]. Noradrenaline increases CBF when acting directly on the cerebral parenchyma after administration into a lateral ventricle or after intracarotid injection combined with osmotic opening of the BBB [197] because of noradrenaline's inability to penetrate the normal BBB [217, 236]. Furthermore, recent studies suggest that reserpine-released central norepinephrine can influence CBF through noradrenergic effects on brain metabolism as shown by changes in glucose uptake and oxygen consumption [189, 199]. The peripheral sympathetic effects of angiotensin have been reviewed by Zimmermann [292].

3. Results

3.1. The Normal Pial Vessels

The characteristic shape of pial vessels has been described by several authors [12]. They are in agreement on all points except intervascular connections.

Arteries and arterioles are conical when observed over a longer distance. They can easily be recognized by this form and their color (Fig. 6). Their diameter is smaller than that of venous vessels and they tend to be less frequent. Arteries course in wide curves (Figs. 6 and 10), dividing less frequently than veins and always in curvilinear form, never in angles. With a few exceptions they tend to run into the cortex vertically after forming a loop which sometimes completes nearly a whole circle (Figs. 6 and 9). The flow within arterial vessels is so rapid that its direction can hardly be distinguished. Slow or stagnant flow was seen extremely rarely in my own experiments. I saw it in only two out of all the animals in interarterial connections [12, 22] (Fig. 6). Schmidt [245—250], Rodda and Denny-Brown [237] described interarterial connections as being frequent and forming a circular network. Interarterial connections were rarely noted in my own material probably owing to the relatively high magnifications which do not allow a survey over a larger brain surface area and especially the border zones between the major arteries.

Venous vessels are greater in number and size. Their shape is cylindrical between single divisions; their diameter changes right at the point of inflow of a branch (Fig. 6). Their course is either irregular or linear rather than curvilinear, as the arterial vessels. The irregularities in venous diameter have been called "sinusoidal" [58], a description that seems somewhat exaggerated except at the point where venous vessels emerge from the cortex into the subarachnoid space.

Venous branching is often rectangular (Fig. 9, see p. 59) but many other kinds of angles are noted (Figs. 6–10). The typical arterial curvilinear course is missing. A frequent observation is narrowing of a branch's diameter right at the point where it enters another venous branch (Fig. 10, see p. 59). Between single branches of venous outflow I could see a great number of intervenous connections in the range below 50 μm, as Florey did [98] (Figs. 6–10). Clark and Wentsler, however, held such intervenous connections to be a rather rare observation [58]. I have included a number of figures in this chapter to demonstrate that these intervenous connections are frequent, as this point will be of importance in a later chapter. Blood flow can easily be observed within smaller venous vessels below 200 μm in diameter. Especially with

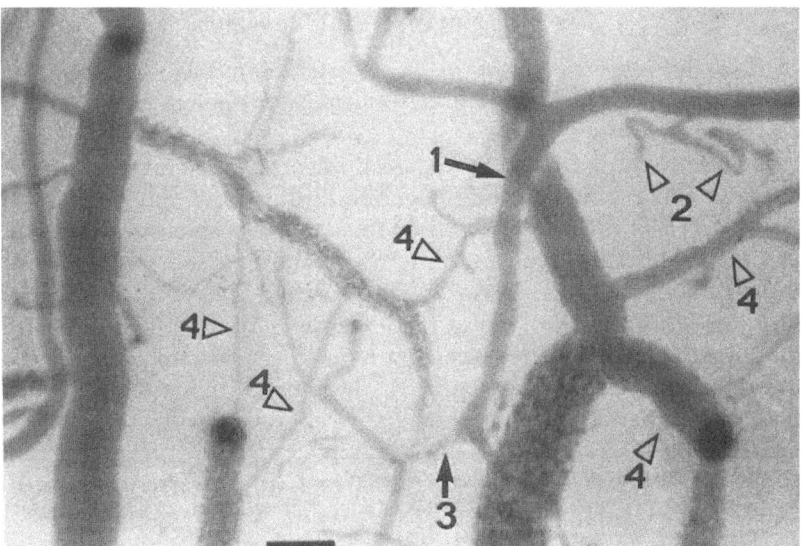

Fig. 6. Normal pial vessels of a cat. Black line = 120 μm. *1* Typical conical shape of arteriole and diffuse staining of the latter due to rapid flow. *2* Small arteriolar branches forming a loop before entering the cortex; *3* One of the rare observations of an interarteriolar connection with slow flow, visible as granular structure of slowly moving blood cells; *4* Intervenous connections. Venules are seen to be more numerous and larger, with different flow speeds in single branches. The branching angles differ widely and are often rectangular. The venous vessels are cylindrical rather than conical and sometimes irregular in diameter. Narrowing at the site of branching is sometimes visible

plasma staining (Evans' blue, sodium fluorescence), the laminar flow becomes visible from the smallest branches to the major branches (Fig. 7). There the blood column is formed by a number of smaller columns, each representing the stream out of a small branch that does not mix with other blood over long distances. Changes in direction of flow occur frequently at the veno-venous connections, where the blood stream often stagnates over longer periods of time. Stagnant flow, however, was never seen to be the cause of thrombosis or even red blood cell agglutination [12] (Fig. 8). A further observation is a column, rich in plasma, which contains a few cells floating in a slow and turbulent stream at the border of the fast-flowing blood in one of the two branches (Fig. 7).

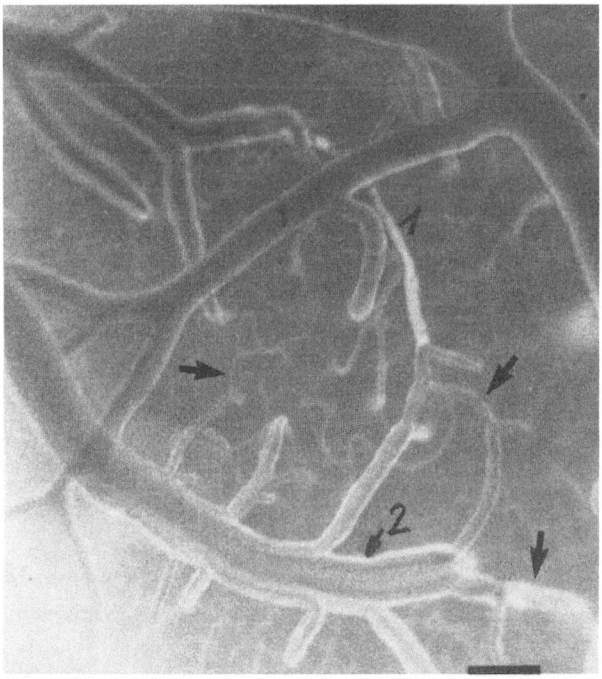

Fig. 7. Fluorescence angiogram of normal pial vessels. Black line = 183 μm. *1* Stagnant plasma in intervenous connection; the arrow indicates other intervenous connection. *2* Typical pattern of laminar flow in larger venule. The blood of an entering branch is seen to force the blood column of the larger vein toward the center; the entering blood remains isolated over a long distance without mixing with the other blood. It is thus easy to determine the direction of flow

Photometrical measurement gives a continuous curve of vessel diameter changes. The characteristics of this curve depend on the objective magnification in use. Using the ultropak 22 or 32, diameter curves of single vessels can be produced. Besides gross changes in diameter, produced by changing blood pressure or blood CO_2 partial pressure (Fig. 11), they show rhythmical changes synchronous with pulse and respiration as well as another biorhythm with a frequency of 2–5 per minute. The latter corresponds well with rhythmical

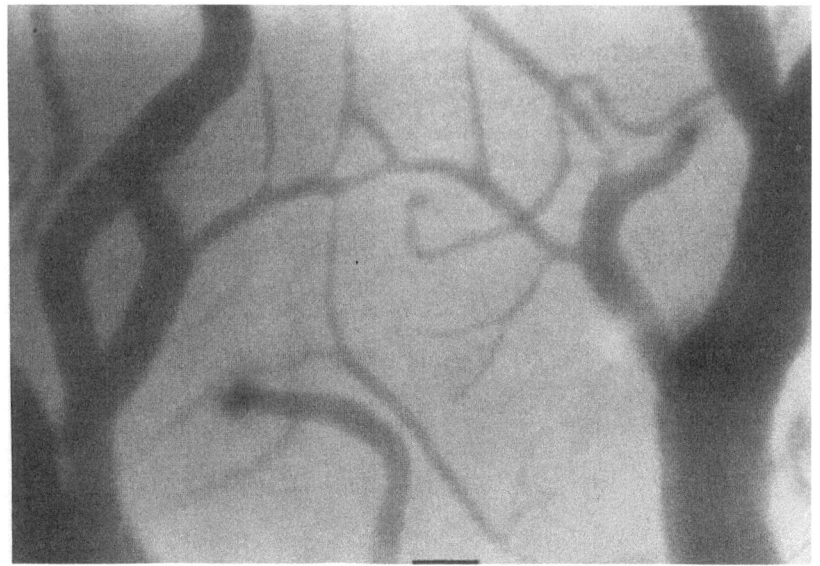

Fig. 8 a

Fig. 8. Normal pial vessels in the cat. Black line = 66 μm. Different flow patterns in a network of intervenous connections. Depending on flow direction and quantity within individual branches, prestasis or stagnant flow occurs in intervenous connections. Flow is restored after varying periods of time without any activation of the coagulatory system or clumping of red blood cells

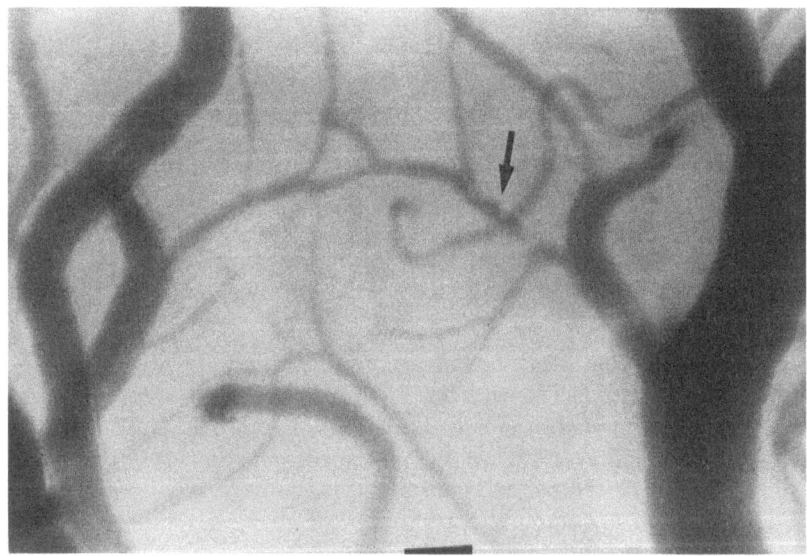

Fig. 8 b

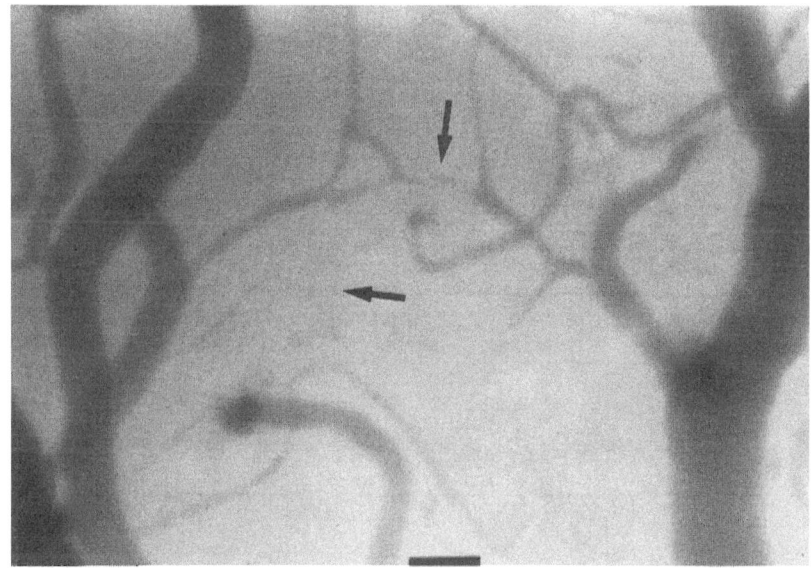

Fig. 8 c

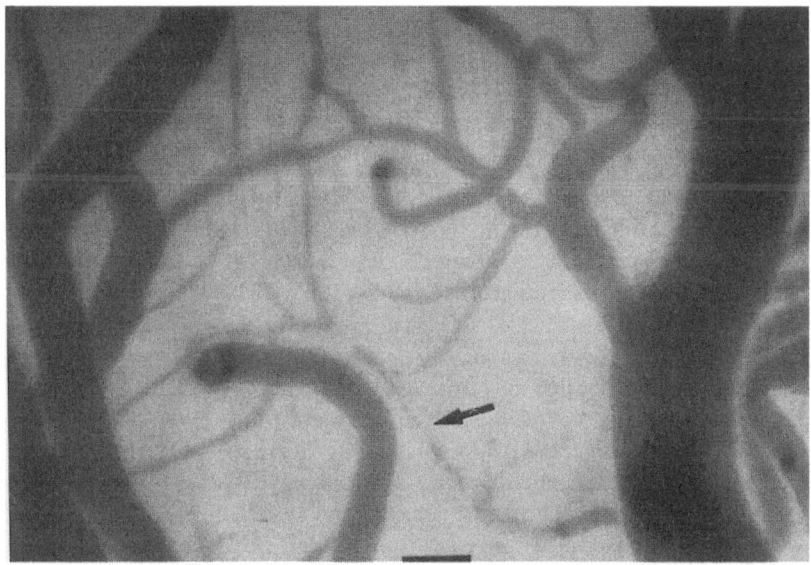

Fig. 8 d

changes in local cerebral blood flow and tissue pO_2, as described by
Severinghaus [254, 255], Moskalenko, Cooper (cit. Severinghaus [255]),
Heuser [141], Clark [59], Betz [35], Lübbers [193], and Leniger-Follert
et al. [190, 191].

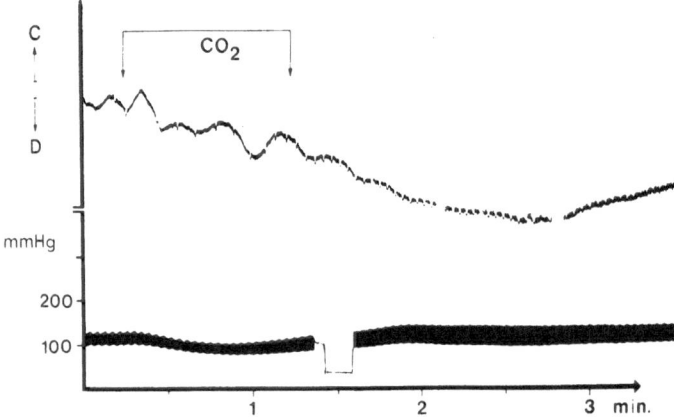

Fig. 11. Lower curve: blood pressure; upper curve: photometric measurement of
the diameter of cat pial vessel. The arrow indicates whether the vessel tends to
constrict (*C*) or dilate (*D*), as the measurements are not scaled. Vasodilatation
during hypercapnia is accompanied by disappearance of the 3–5 per minute
oscillations. Arrow indicates beginning of CO_2 inhalation

3.2. Pial Arteriolar Diameter Changes During Hypertension

3.2.1. Hypertension During Normocapnia and Normal pH

I wanted to test the hypothesis that a sudden and high (on
percentage basis) increase in blood pressure leads to cerebrovascular
lesions. I wished also to ascertain whether there could be another
decisive factor unrelated to arterial pressure. The aim of the intravital microscopic study was to relate pial arteriolar diameter changes
and certain characteristics of the arterial pressure increase such as
steepness of the pressor response and percentage increase in MABP.
Experiments were performed in two groups of animals with different
periods for the arterial pressure increase [21]. This was achieved by
using the drugs described in the "Methods" chapter. Furthermore,
the influence of hyper- and hypocapnia as well as metabolic acidosis
and alkalosis was studied so as to understand how metabolic changes
could modulate the upper limit of autoregulation. In a third experimental group, differing vascular reaction patterns were distinguished,
dependent on different blood-pressure characteristics, by photometry.

Group 1:

Blood Pressure

After the injection of Hypertensin®, MABP rose within 20 to 120 seconds (mean 58 seconds) from 70—150 mm Hg (mean 110.59 mm Hg) to 170–225 mm Hg (mean 208.12 mm Hg). Percentage increase ranged from + 40% to + 200% over the resting values (mean 93.88%). Single results are given in Table 4.

Table 4

Group 1								
MABP				**Time**		**Gas-check**		
Exp.	Resting value mm Hg	Peak value mm Hg	%	MABP-increase within seconds	MABP return to resting value within minutes	P_aCO_2	pH	P_aO_2
F 26	150	210	+ 40	32	3	58	7.20	121
F 36	150	255	+ 70	90	5	35	7.37	155
F 37	100	193	+ 93	30	9	54	7.15	103
F 38	70	210	+ 200	60	11	42	7.35	166
F 39	110	175	+ 59	60	4	38	7.37	119
F 40	90	190	+ 111	30	—	40	7.49	158
F 41	105	205	+ 95	90	12	46	7.30	114
F 46	150	250	+ 67	50	5	36	7.39	200
F 47	120	220	+ 83	40	4.5	43	7.40	177
F 48	105	210	+ 100	45	—	35	7.36	143
F 50	115	190	+ 65	30	6	42	7.37	115
F 51	80	170	+ 113	20	> 5	25	7.44	143
F 52	120	200	+ 66	60	5	36	7.37	144
F 53	95	210	+ 121	90	5	35	7.36	187
F 56	115	210	+ 83	42	5	27	7.44	172
F 58	110	230	+ 109	90	5	44	7.37	148
F 59	95	210	+ 121	120	> 5	27	7.45	171

Blood Gases

In ten animals, P_aCO_2 remained within 35–44 mm Hg (mean 38.6 mm Hg), pH between 7.35 and 7.40 (mean 7.371), P_aO_2 between 115 and 200 mm Hg (mean 155.4 mm Hg) (see Table 4). The values of hypo- and hypercapnic and alkalotic animals immediately before the onset of hypertension are also given in Table 4. Hypercapnia was between 46 and 58 mm Hg, hypocapnia between 25 and 17 mm Hg.

Reactions of Arterial Vessels

Arterial dilatation in this group frequently showed a latency of up to 1 minute or more. The most common reaction was initial constriction during the increase in arterial pressure and during the pressure plateau (see Fig. 12). On vessels $\leq$ 30 µm in resting diameter, the constriction was — 21.6% at 30 seconds. After 60 seconds—when, on the average, the pressure plateau had been reached—the dilatation was still less than + 10% (mean). It was only after 120 seconds, when the mean dilatation, ranging from — 7% to

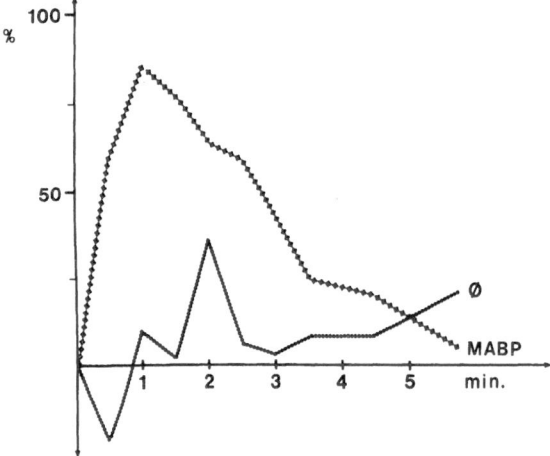

Fig. 12. Percentage comparison of mean arterial vessel diameter ($\varnothing$) and MABP changes during the first 5 minutes after onset of acute hypertension. Vessels up to 30 µm resting diameter in group 1

+ 88%, was + 36%. Thereafter vessel caliber returned to + 10% (Fig. 12). These relatively low values for mean arterial vessel dilatation conceal widely differing types of vascular reactions in the cats in this group, as presented in Table 5, where single measurements are given. In one and the same cat, diffuse dilatation and constriction could be seen in different vessels, as well as sausage-like dilatation with interposed narrow segments. A further pattern was that sometimes there was an initial, slight dilatation with a subsequent marked constriction as in normal autoregulatory responses. On the other hand, diffuse constriction could occur at the beginning of the pressure rise and remain for a few minutes until, finally, segmental or diffuse dilatation broke through, which continued even after the 5 minutes during which arterial pressure returned to its resting value (Fig. 13). Single measurements of maximum dilatation or constriction during

Table 5. *Degrees of Dilation in Group 1*

Resting diameter up to 30 μm				Resting diameter above 30 μm			
Exp.	Resting diameter μm	Peak diameter μm	%	Exp.	Resting diameter μm	Peak diameter μm	%
F 36	16.5	31.6	+ 112.5	F 37 A	45	51	+ 13
F 37	30	51	+ 70	B	48	57	+ 19
F 36 A	27	34.5	+ 27	C	52.5	60	+ 14
B	25.5	28.5	+ 6	D	33	40.5	+ 23
C	21	25.5	+ 21	F 36 K	33	93	+ 177
D	31.5	76.5	+ 138	F 38 B	200	205	+ 3
H	28.5	75	+ 163	C	210	285	+ 83
L	10.5	34.5	+ 229	D	200	250	+ 25
M	4.5	6	+ 33	F	40	55	+ 38
O	10.5	43.5	+ 286	G	60	70	+ 17
Q	6.75	9	+ 33	F 46 A	35	45	+ 28.6
R	4.5	6	+ 33	F 47 A	105	155	+ 48
S	4.5	6	+ 33	L	42	102	+ 183
T	4.5	36	+ 380	F 48 A	62.5	—	—
F 48 C	30	35	+ 17	B	47.5	50	+ 5
E	27.5	32.5	+ 18	E	52.5	11	+ 5
G	27.5	35	+ 27	F 52 C	32.5	65	+ 100
H	12.5	17.5	+ 40	A	87.5	92.5	+ 6
F 52 D	27.5	40	+ 45	F 53 A	77.5	125	+ 61
E	15	20	+ 33	B	82.5	125	+ 52
F	17.5	20	+ 14	E	75	87.5	+ 17
O	5	10	+ 100	F	77.5	95	+ 23
F 53 C	15	22.5	+ 50	M	70	115	+ 64
D	15	15	—				
G	12.5	17.5	+ 40				
H	10	15	+ 50				
Q	10	—	—				
R	7.5	5	− 33				

the first 5 minutes are given in Table 5 and show the trend of vascular reactions in those experiments in which break-through was noted. Although there is a wide range of differing reactions, the graphic demonstration in Fig. 14 shows the tendency of smaller vessels to react more markedly than larger ones.

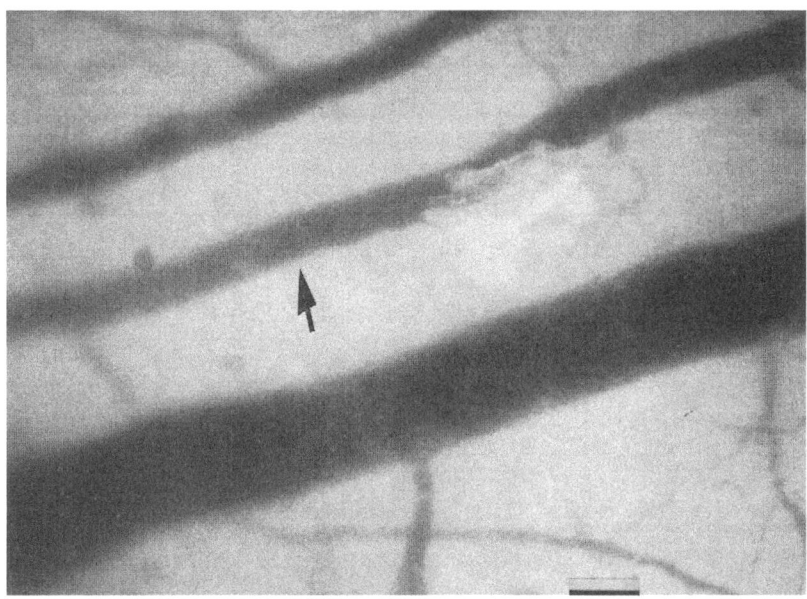

Fig. 13 a. Normal pial vessels before hypertension. MABP = 120 mm Hg. Arrow indicates arteriole; black line = 183 μm

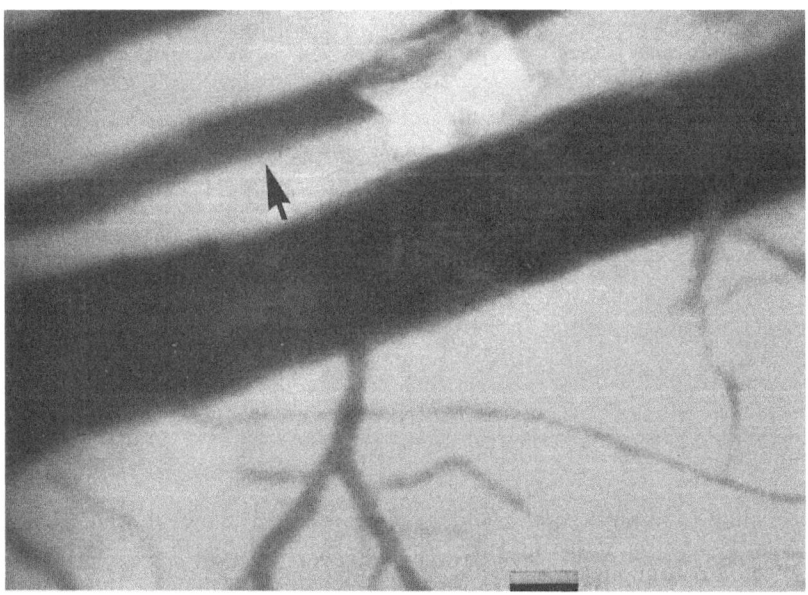

Fig. 13 b. 2.5 minutes later marked venous dilatation is seen along with unchanged arterioles. MABP = 220 mm Hg

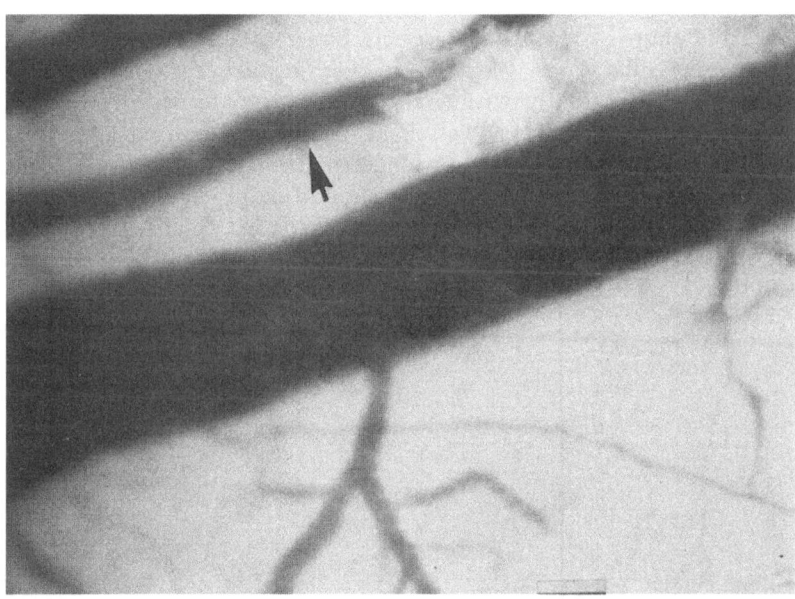

Fig. 13 c. At 3.5 minutes and an MABP of 140 mm Hg, arterial vessels begin to dilate

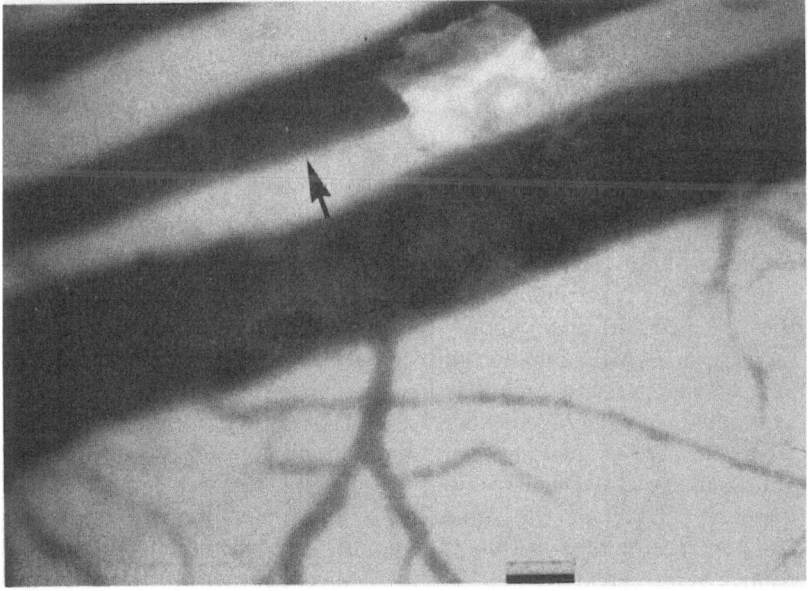

Fig. 13 d. The same site 4.5 minutes after beginning of hypertension and an MABP of 120 mm Hg. The arteriole is extremely dilated

Segmental dilatation, the so-called "sausage-string" phenomenon occurred more frequently in vessels under 30 μm resting diameter. Segmental dilatations occurred in varying lengths and numbers, sometimes individually within a general pattern of diffuse constriction. The "sausage-string" vessels nearly always changed their form, the dilated segments becoming longer or shorter, thicker or thinner, within a few minutes. This phenomenon often began close to bifurcations. As seen in Fig. 14, dilatation ranged from + 63% to + 400% in these segments of vessels ≤ 30 μm, *i.e.*, a five-fold increase from

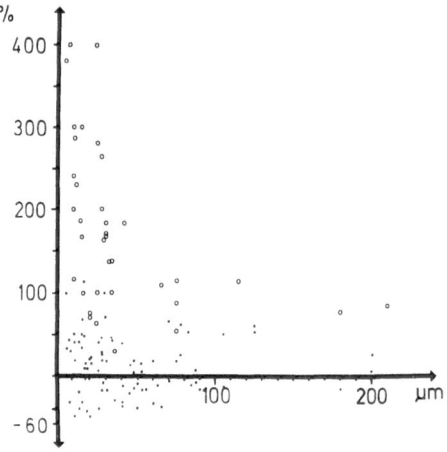

Fig. 14. Resting diameters of arterial vessels in group 1 plotted against percentage increase during hypertension. Dots: diameter changes without sausage-like deformations. Circles: measurements on sausages. Although there is a very wide range of reactions from marked constriction to extreme dilatation, it can be seen that small vessels dilate and constrict more than larger vessels, and that the function is not linear but curvilinear

resting values (mean + 99%). Comparing blood-pressure characteristics with the type and extent of arterial vessel diameter changes, they seemed—in this group—to depend firstly on the percentage increase in MABP, and secondly on its peak value, with the acuteness of the pressure increase the least important. Fig. 15 gives an example of a 65% MABP increase to 190 mm Hg within 30 seconds, where the short "sausages" were noted despite most vessels displaying autoregulatory vasoconstriction. In Fig. 16 the percentage MABP increase was about the same (67%); but the pressure peak was 250 mm Hg, reached within 50 seconds, and the number of dilated segments was greater. Fig. 17 shows an experiment with 121% increase in MABP to 210 mm Hg within 90 seconds, where multiple sausages occurred.

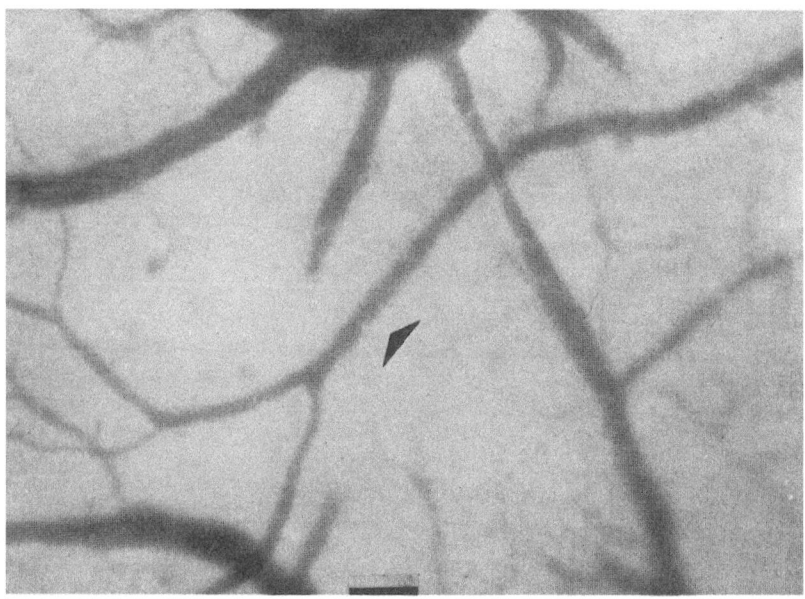

Fig. 15 a. Normal pial vessels before hypertension. Arrow indicates arteriole.
Black line = 183 μm; MABP = 115 mm Hg

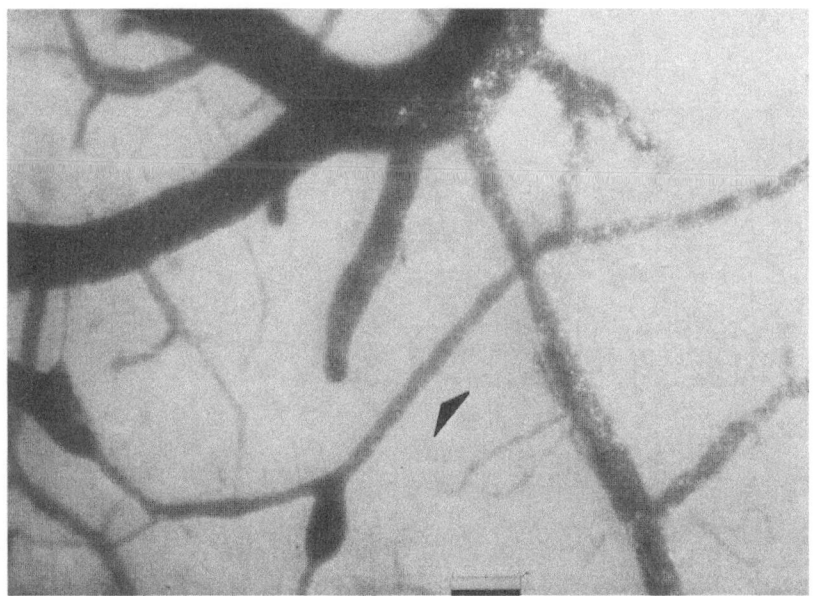

Fig. 15 b. Two minutes after onset of hypertension; MABP = 190 mm Hg

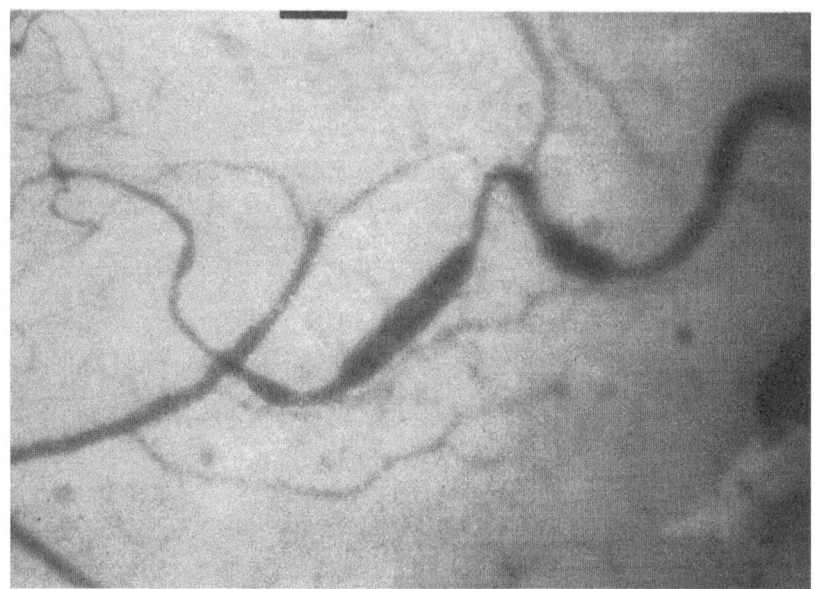

Fig. 16. A section of the region observed before onset of hypertension. Several sausages developed after 2.5 minutes at an MABP of 200 mm Hg. Black line = 183 µm

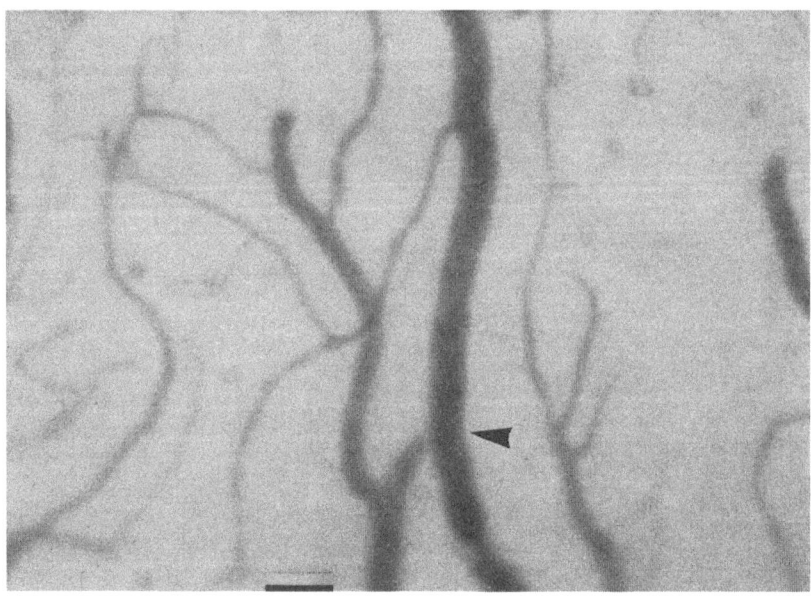

Fig. 17 a. Normal situation of pial vessels at MABP of 120 mm Hg. Arrow indicates arteriole with branches. Black line = 183 µm

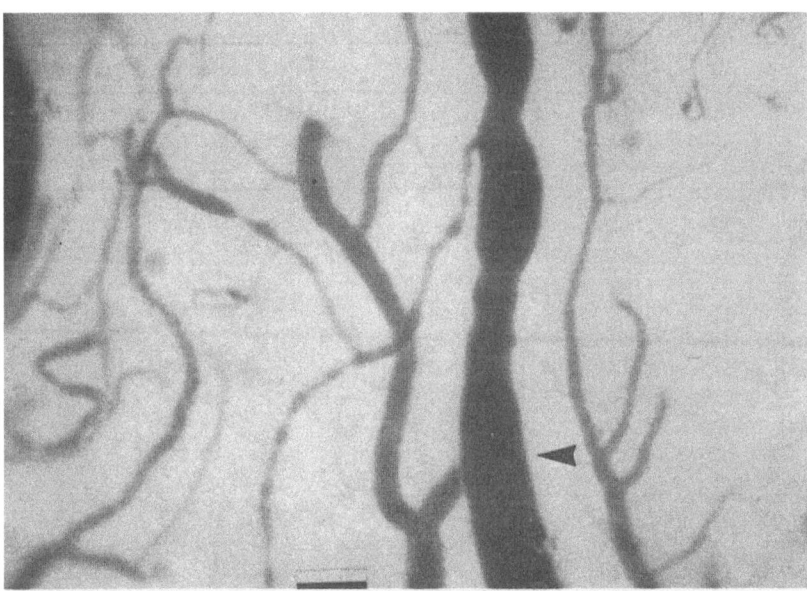

Fig. 17 b. Multiple sausage-like dilatations are still present after 12 minutes at MABP = 120 mm Hg. Black line = 183 µm

Group 2:

Blood Pressure

This series of experiments was designed to examine the more pronounced vascular effects of extremely acute hypertension. Here the MABP increase occurred within 9–30 seconds (mean 20.2 seconds) in the five normocapnic cats which were comparable with group 1 (Table 6 B). Pressure rose from 60–125 mm Hg (mean 98 mm Hg) to 150–250 mm Hg (mean 210 mm Hg). The percentage increase varied from + 83.3 to 167 (mean value 121.8%). MABP plateaued for 1.2–4 minutes and returned to resting values within 4.5–14 minutes. Two cats were excluded from comparison with group 1 (Table 6 A) because the pressor response was small and the latency was fairly considerable.

Blood Gases and pH

In the course of the experiments, P_aCO_2 remained between 30 and 44 mm Hg, pH 7.30–7.44, P_aO_2 74–118, in five animals

Table 6. *Group 2 and 3*

MABP					Time			Gas-check		
	Exp.	Resting value mm Hg	Peak value mm Hg	%	Increase to peak seconds	Plateau minutes	Return to rest. minutes	P_aCO_2	pH	P_aO_2
A	F 64	120	180	+ 50	120	4	14	44	7.30	108
	F 65	100	160	+ 60	62	3	7.5	32	7.36	109
B	F 67	60	150	+ 150	20	15	—	30	7.35	106
	F 68	110	230	+ 109	24	2	9	37	7.34	91
	F 69	120	220	+ 83.3	30	1.2	8	43	7.39	118
	F 75/I	125	250	+ 100	18	2.5	—	41	7.33	74
	F 75/III	75	200	+ 167	9	2.5	—	37	7.44	92
C	F 73	100	175	+ 75	24	2	—	41	7.50	115
	F 74	75	200	+ 166.6	9	1.5	12	30	7.59	106
D	P 2	150	240	+ 60	18	1	14	37	7.35	100
	P 3	120	180	+ 50	5	1	4	33	7.40	112
	P 4	70	150	+ 114.3	15	—	—	27	7.46	124
	P 5	90	150	+ 66.7	6	—	—	42	7.38	130
	P 6	130	230	+ 76.9	15	—	—	30	7.38	105
	P 7	100	150	+ 50	8	—	—	21	7.42	150

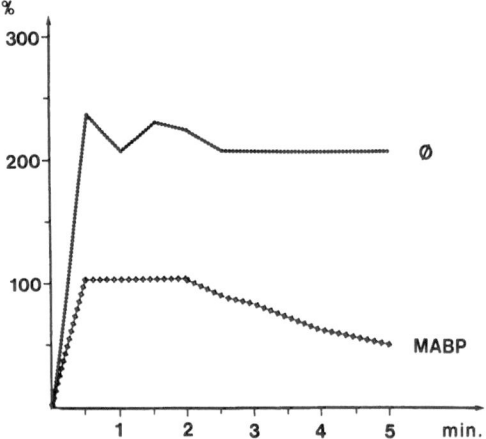

Fig. 18. Percentage comparison of mean arterial vessel diameter ($\varnothing$) and MABP changes during the first 5 minutes after onset of acute hypertension. Vessels ≤ 30 μm resting diameter in group 2

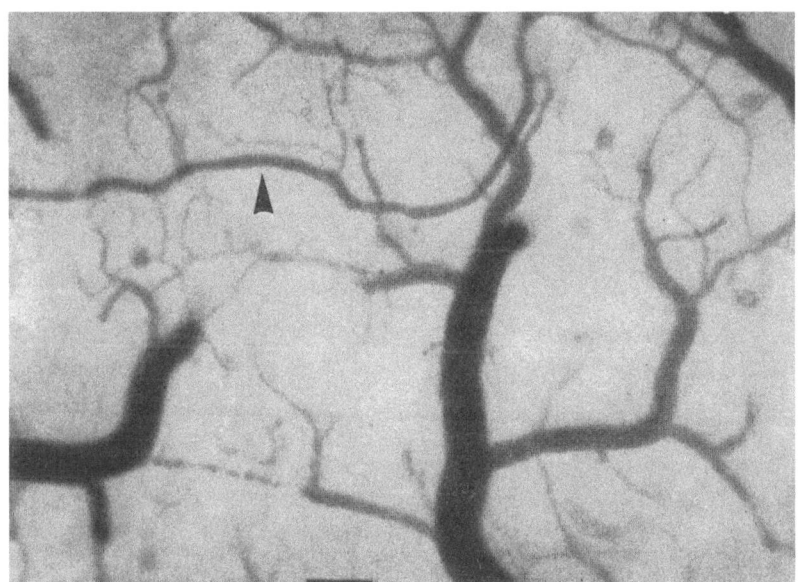

Fig. 19 a. Normal situation of pial vessels before hypertension. MABP 110 mm Hg.
Arrow indicates arteriole with branches. Black line = 183 μm

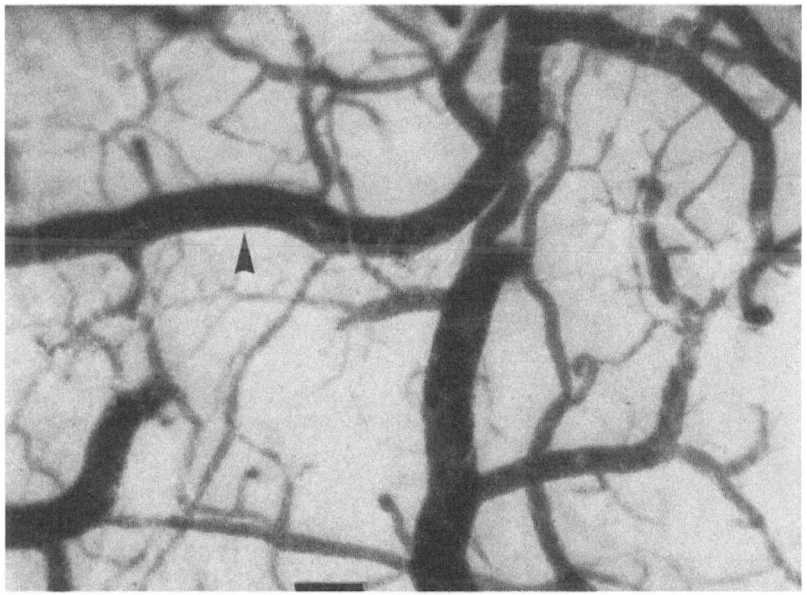

Fig. 19 b. MABP increase to 230 mm Hg was produced within 24 seconds. The
situation shown in the picture is at an MABP of 160 mm Hg 4.5 minutes after
onset of hypertension. Venous dilatation is evident, yet less marked than arteriolar
distension. Black line = 183 μm

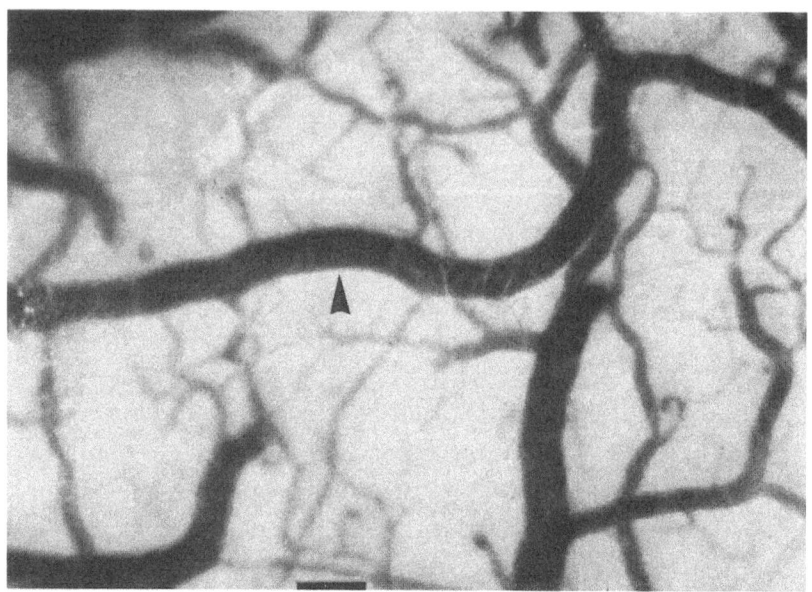

Fig. 19 c. MABP = 100 mm Hg, 10 minutes after beginning of hypertension. There is still extreme diffuse vasodilatation. Black line = 183 μm

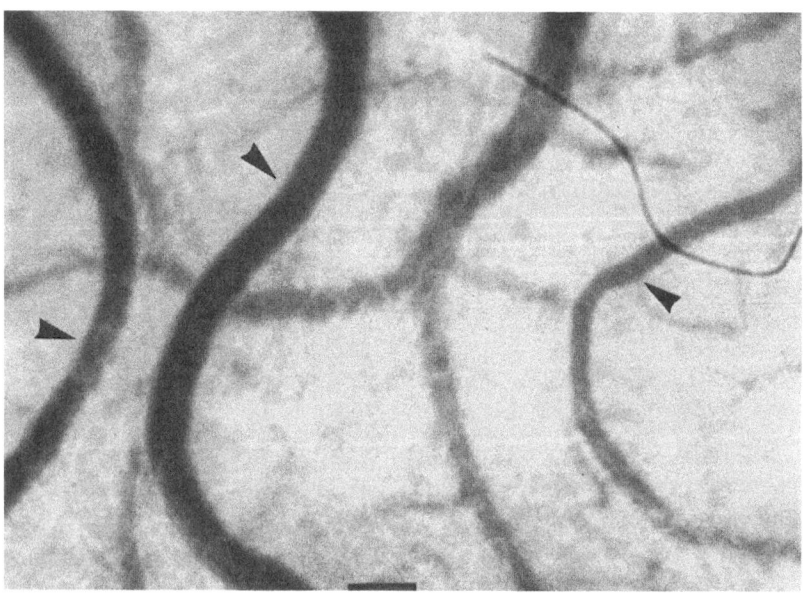

Fig. 20 a. Normal situation before hypertension. MABP 70 mm Hg. Arrow shows three arterioles. Fibers of preserved arachnoid membrane are visible. Black line = 183 μm

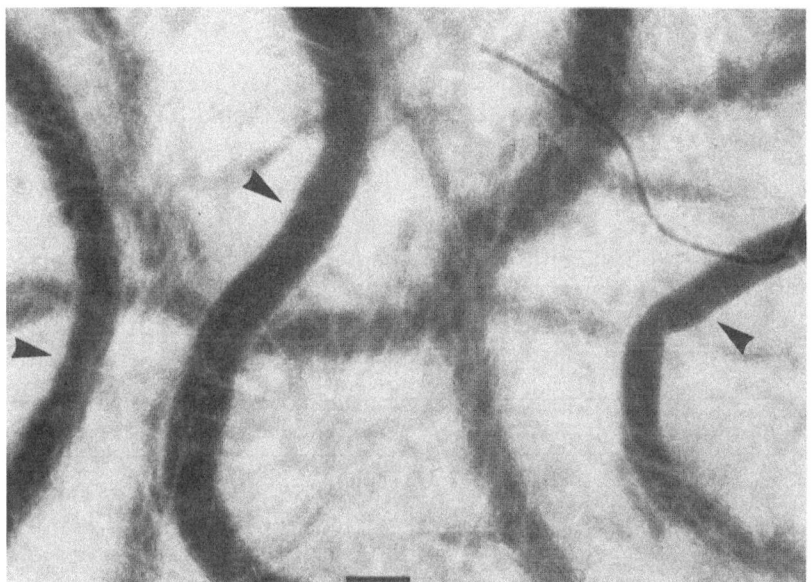

Fig. 20 b. Acute hypertension occurring within 20 seconds (MABP = 150 mm Hg). Diffuse vasodilatation, only one short narrow segment, reddening of venules. Black line = 183 μm

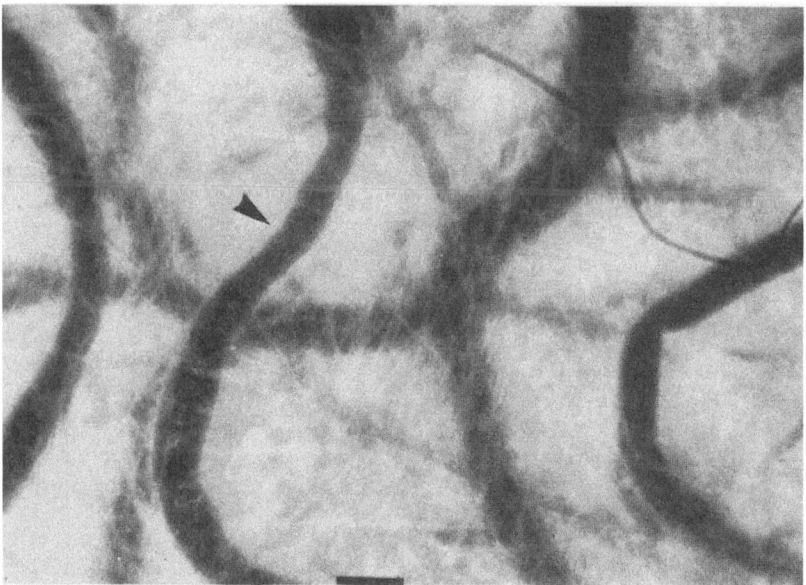

Fig. 20 c. After 2 minutes, the diffuse type of arteriolar dilatation has changed to a sausage-like dilatation with narrow segments visible in the center of the picture (arrow)

(Table 6 B). In two animals, metabolic alkalosis occurred with pH between 7.50 and 7.59 and $[HCO_3]^-$ of 32.3 and 33.0 meq/l (see Table 6 C).

Arterial Vessel Reactions

In the two cats with a slow response and a low percentage pressure increase, no marked dilatation was visible. Pronounced dilata-

Table 7. *Diameter Changes of Group 2*

Resting diameter up to 30 μm				Resting diameter above 30 μm			
Exp.	Resting diameter μm	Peak diameter μm	%	Exp.	Resting diameter μm	Peak diameter μm	%
F 68 A	25	100	+ 300	F 67 A	80	110	+ 37.5
B	20	100	+ 400	B	85	115	+ 35.3
C	7.5	45	+ 500	C	100	135	+ 35
D	22.5	95	+ 322	D	100	130	+ 30
E	25	100	+ 300	E	95	125	+ 31.6
F	12.5	90	+ 620	F	50	95	+ 90
G	10	60	+ 500	G	50	80	+ 60
H	10	45	+ 350	H	55	105	+ 91
K	10	50	+ 400	F 69 C	35	100	+ 185.7
L	10	35	+ 250	D	35	125	+ 257.1
M	10	30	+ 200	F	35	110	+ 214.3
F 69 A	30	100	+ 233	G	40	110	+ 175
B	30	95	+ 217	H	35	135	+ 285.7
E	20	65	+ 225	N	35	85	+ 143
K	20	55	+ 175	F 75/I A	50	60	+ 20
L	15	70	+ 267	B	35	45	+ 29
F 75/I G	15	20	+ 33	C	35	45	+ 29
F 75/III P	30	75	+ 150	D	40	50	+ 25
F 75/III R	15	35	+ 133	E	30	50	+ 67
S	10	35	+ 250	H	215	265	+ 21
F 75/I F	25	35	+ 40	K	130	170	+ 35
F 75/III G	100	135	+ 35	L	145	175	+ 21
H	95	140	+ 47	M	145	170	+ 17
K	100	135	+ 35	N	85	100	+ 35
L	45	80	+ 78	O	105	115	+ 10
M	35	85	+ 143	F 75/III A	60	95	+ 58
N	40	70	+ 75	B	70	100	+ 43
O	40	75	+ 88	C	105	160	+ 52
Q	65	130	+ 100	D	110	175	+ 59
				E	110	160	+ 40
				F	95	240	+ 153

tion and constriction could be seen in one cat together with venous dilatation, similar to the results in group 1. In five animals, however, with a pressure increase of more than 80% (Table 6 B), diffuse arteriolar dilatation was found and, on average, was maximal after 30 seconds (Fig. 18). In two cats the arterioles distended most suddenly during the peak of the pressor wave; it seemed as if the vessels would burst at any moment. This state of maximal distension continued for more than 5 minutes (Fig. 19) in those two cats and then the state changed to one of segmental dilatation after 2 minutes in one cat (Fig. 20), a state which remained for more than 10 min-

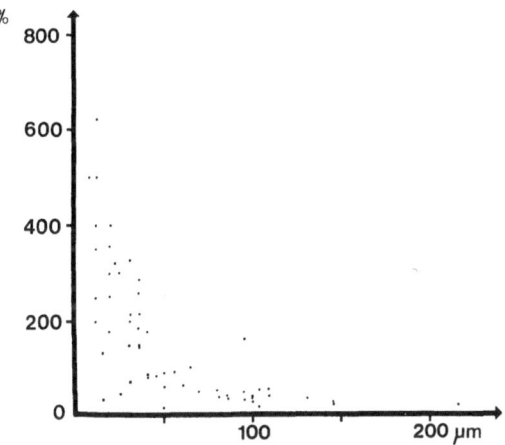

Fig. 21. Arterial resting diameters of group 2 plotted against percentage diameter increase during hypertension. The curvilinear relationship is readily apparent

utes. Arterial vessels under 30 μm resting diameter (7.5–30 μm, mean 17.34 μm) dilated to 30–100 μm, mean 70.94 μm. The percentage increase in caliber ranged from + 175 to + 620 and was + 341.19 on average.

Arterioles over 30 μm (35–100 μm) dilated to 80–135 μm (mean 111.4 μm). The percentage increase varied between + 30% and + 285.7%, mean 119.4%, which is twice normal. Individual results are given in Table 7. When these results are plotted against the resting diameters, a clear cross correlation (Fig. 21) between resting diameter and percentage dilatation becomes visible which is similar to the exponential curve [23] that was observed during hypercapnia. In comparison to the normocapnic cats in group 1, vasodilatation was much more impressive, occurred signif-

< 30 µm

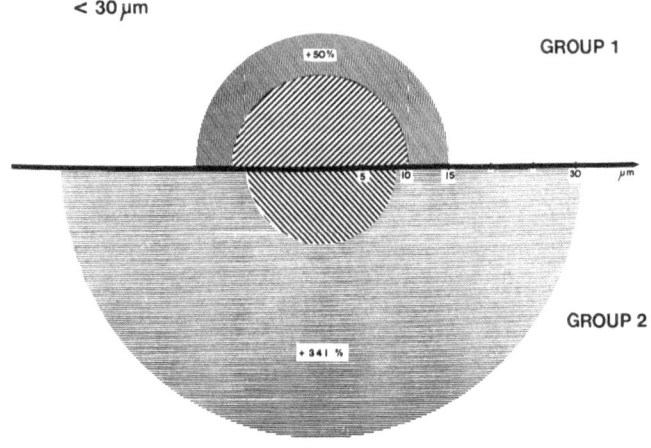

Fig. 22 a

> 30 µm

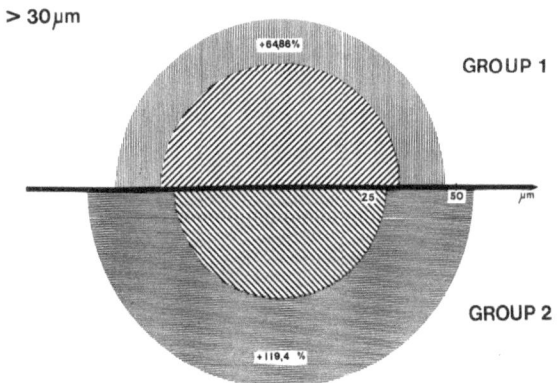

Fig. 22 b

Fig. 22. Comparison of mean arterial diameter changes in group 1 (upper halves) and group 2 (lower halves). It may be seen that the vessels in group 2 dilate more than those in group 1. a) Vessels ≤ 30 µm; b) vessels > than 30 µm. The differing reactions of smaller and larger vessels can be seen only in group 2. In group 1, constriction accompanying dilatation obscures the true dilatation values (see Fig. 12)

icantly faster and remained markedly longer in group 2 (see Fig. 22). When comparing the pressure response characteristics of both groups (see Figs. 17 and 18), it can be seen clearly that arterial pressure reached its peak within about half the time in group 2, while percentage increase and the absolute value for the pressure peak were generally similar.

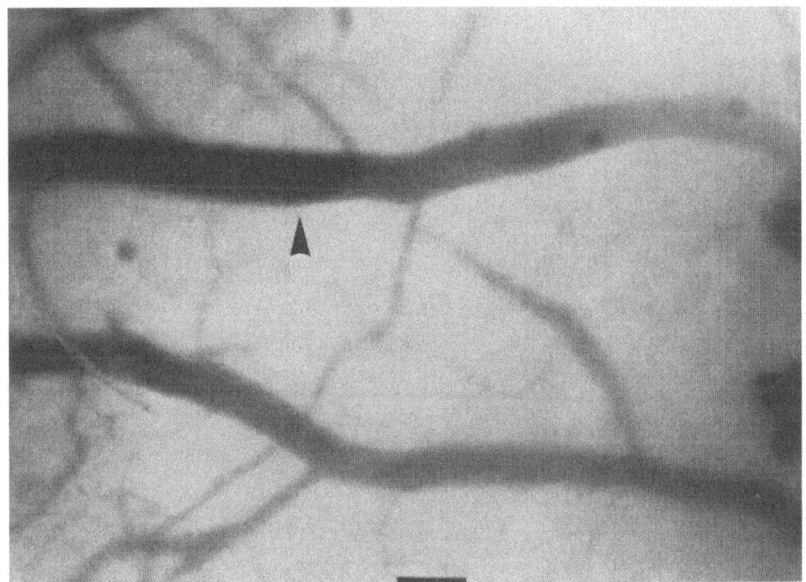

Fig. 23 a. Pial vessels at MABP of 150 mm Hg, P_aCO_2 58 mm Hg, pH 7.20 immediately before onset of acute hypertension. Arrow indicates arteriole. Black line = 183 μm

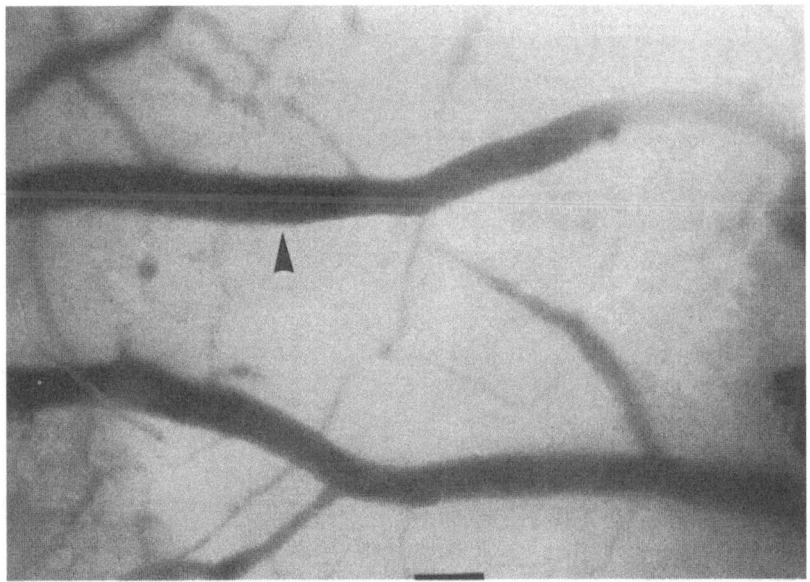

Fig. 23 b. Three minutes after beginning of hypertension and return of MABP to 160 mm Hg, the arterioles show diffuse but sharp constriction. No signs of break-trough

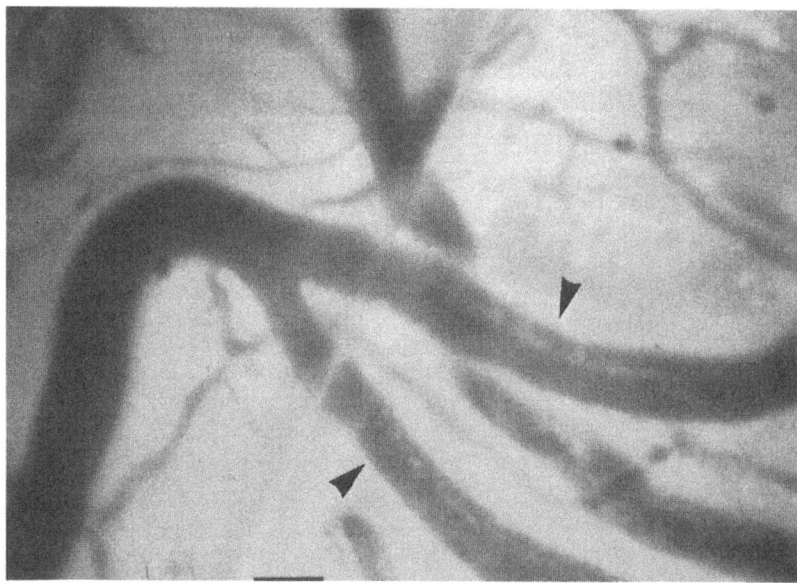

Fig. 24 a. Pial vessels at P_aCO_2 64 mm Hg and pH 7.30 immediately before hypertension. Arrow indicates arterioles. Black line = 65 μm, MABP = 105 mm Hg

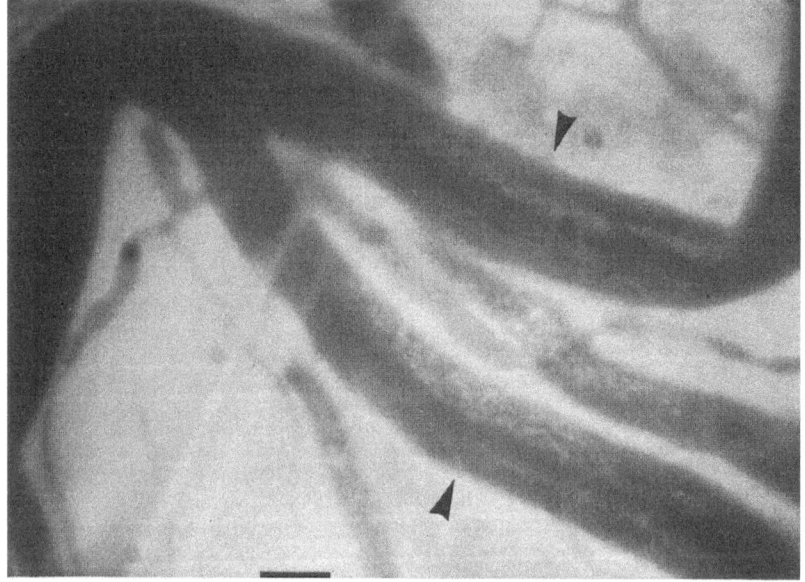

Fig. 24 b. Extreme vasodilatation as long as 7 minutes after onset of hypertension. MABP 140 mm Hg. Black line = 66 μm

3.2.2. Hypertension During Metabolic Acidosis and Hypercapnia

This situation was produced in three animals in group 1. In one animal (Table 4, F 26), autoregulation remained intact during a blood-pressure increase of 40% to MABP of 210 mm Hg (Fig. 23). One animal (Table 4, F 37) with P_aCO_2 of 54 and pH 7.15 showed a blood-pressure increase of 93%. Diffuse vasodilatation was seen for somewhat more than 60 seconds, during the slow return to normal BP. There was, however, no extreme distension with formation of sausages. The third animal (Table 4, F 41) had nearly normal values with a P_aCO_2 of 46 mm Hg and a pH of 7.30. In this case extreme arteriolar distension developed parallel to the increase in MABP (105 to 205 within 90 seconds) and persisted for more than 10 minutes (Fig. 24).

3.2.3. Hypertension During Hypocapnia

This situation was produced in five animals, three animals of group 1 and two of group 3 (see below). There was dilatation in two cases in group 1, one with a P_aCO_2 of 25 mm Hg (F 51), the other with 27 mm Hg (F 56, F 59). The extent of dilatation and formation of sausages was the same in the two hypocapnic animals as in the normocapnic animals of the group. In the third animal, which also had a P_aCO_2 of 27 mm Hg, autoregulation remained normal and minimal constriction occurred during hypertension; the slow blood-pressure increase may be seen in Table 4.

3.2.4. Hypertension During Metabolic Alkalosis

Metabolic alkalosis was produced in three animals, one in group 1 and two in group 2. One animal (F 40) had a percentage blood-pressure increase of 111% within 30 seconds during a pH of 7.49, P_aCO_2 40 mm Hg and HCO_3^- of 32.2 meq/l, but the arterioles constricted diffusely as they do with normal autoregulation. Only mild venous dilatation and acceleration of flow speed indicated a short phase of somewhat increased blood flow. In the second animal (Table 6, F 73) hypertension was started at a pH of 7.50 and HCO_3^- of 32.3 meq/, P_aCO_2 41 mm Hg. The changes in pial vessels were the same as in the first experiment. The third animal (Table 6, F 74, Table 7) had the highest percentage blood-pressure increase (+ 167%) within 9 seconds. Venous dilatation began after 5 seconds and marked arterial dilatation with formation of sausages occurred after 30 seconds (Fig. 25).

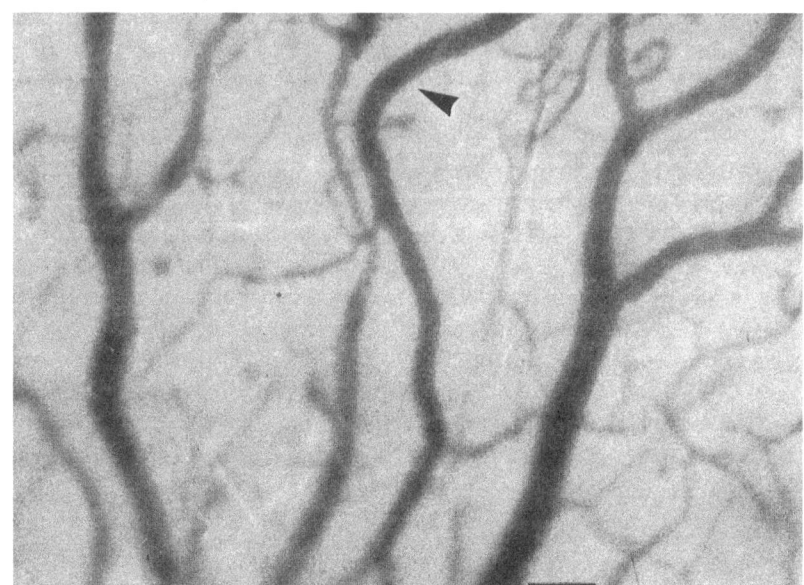

Fig. 25 a. The state of pial vessels at P_aCO_2 30 mm Hg, pH 7.59, MABP 75 mm Hg. Arrow shows arteriole. Black line = 183 μm

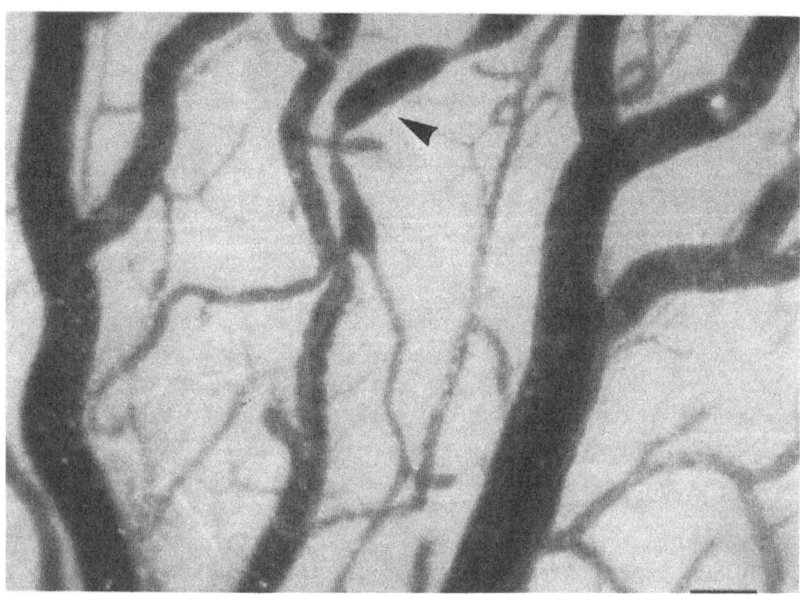

Fig. 25 b. Two and a half minutes after very abrupt onset of severe hypertension (see Table 6, F 74), venous dilatation and formation of arterial sausages with narrow segments and narrow branches are visible. MABP = 200 mm Hg. Black line = 183 μm

In control animals, arterial diameters did not change significantly under normocapnic conditions. They measured up to $\pm$ 0.83%; the same measurements have been reported by other authors [196].

3.2.5. Photometric Results (Group 3)

Four of six animals were normocapnic during the experiments, two hypocapnic. MABP rose from 70–150 mm Hg (see Table 6) (mean 110 mm Hg) to 150–240 mm Hg (mean 183.3 mm Hg), which equals a percentage increase of 50–114% (mean 69.7%). Breakthrough of autoregulation occurred three times (Table 6: P 2, P 4, P 6), in two normocapnic and one hypocapnic animal. MABP was increased to 230 and 240 mm Hg, respectively, the percentage increase was more than + 100%. Signs of vasodilatation appeared immediately with the increase in blood pressure (Fig. 26). Vasodilatation was seen during the whole period of pressure increase and pressure plateau and persisted for 5.5 to 14.5 minutes, after blood pressure had returned to normal or nearly normal. Vascular diameters returned to resting values after more than 20 minutes. Another type of vascular dilatational reaction is shown in Fig. 27. When

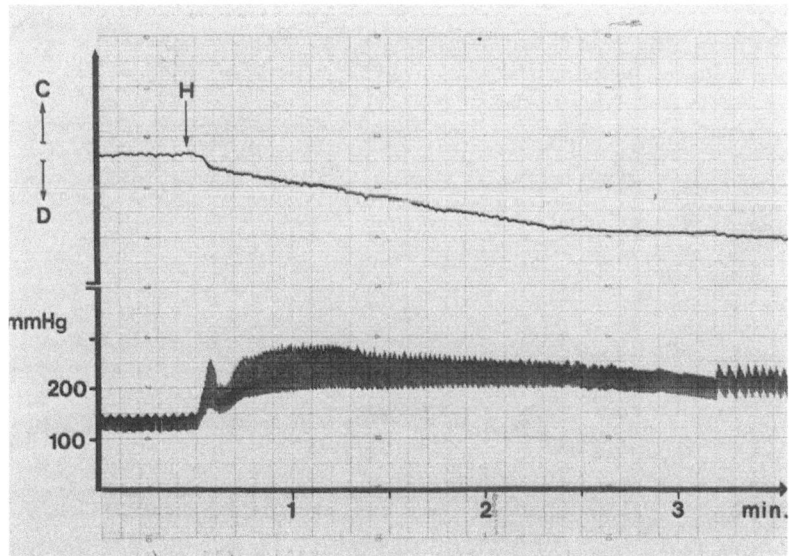

Fig. 26. Lower curve: MABP during the first 3 minutes of acute hypertension. Upper curve: photometrical curve of vascular diameter changes during this period. A falling curve indicates vasodilatation (D), a rising curve vasoconstriction (C). H injection of norepinephrine

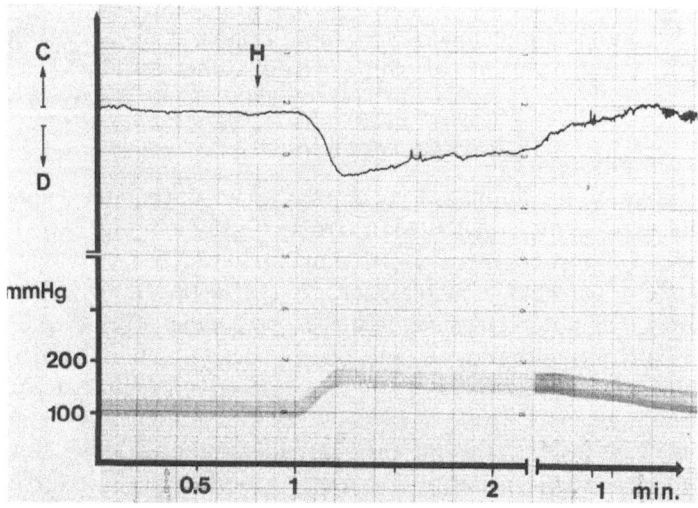

Fig. 27. Lower curve: MABP during the first 9 minutes of hypertension. Upper curve: photometrical curve, showing vasodilatation (D) as a drop in the curve, accompanying the onset of hypertension. At the lowest point of the curve, diffuse arteriolar dilatation without sausages was seen microscopically. Vascular diameters normalized within 5 minutes. H injection of norepinephrine

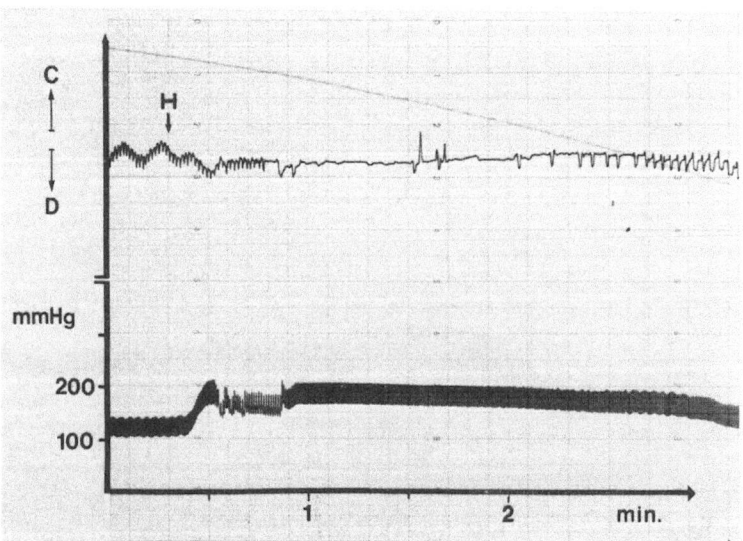

Fig. 28. Lower curve: MABP during the first 3 minutes of acute hypertension. Upper curve: photometrical curve during this time. D vasodilatation, C vasoconstriction, H injection of norepinephrine. The curve did not change; vasodilatation was not observed microscopically

autoregulation was preserved, the photometric extinction curve remained at its resting level, but the small rhythmical changes disappeared for a time (Fig. 28). The percentage blood-pressure increase in these animals under normocapnic conditions was low (Table 6, P 3, P 5), the MABP peak remaining below 200 mm Hg. In this series hypocapnia had no protective effect, with one animal showing severe vasodilatation due to an abrupt, high-percentage MABP increase, and the other remaining without signs of marked dilatation, with an MABP increase of 50%, from 100 to 150 mm Hg within 8 seconds.

3.2.6. The Sausage-String Phenomenon

Results for the estimation of sausages were obtained from animals of group 1 and the slow-increase experiments of group 2. Blood-pressure changes may be seen there. The sausage-string phenomenon was seen in eight out of ten normocapnic cats with neutral blood pH. Arterial diameter changes varied widely without a clear correlation between blood-pressure peak and the extent of vascular changes [17]. Initial diffuse constriction with subsequent diffuse dilatation or segmental dilatation (sausages) was seen, as well as initial diffuse dilatation and subsequent constriction, often followed by formation of some sausages. Segmental and diffuse dilatation variously persisted even as blood pressure returned to its resting value, or diminished to normal or subnormal values when the MABP was still over 200 mm Hg. One example of a few shortlived sausages with interposed constricted areas is shown in Fig. 15. Measurements on 24 sausages produced the results shown in Table 8. Sausages were most frequently seen on arterioles with a resting diameter of less than 30 μm. Sometimes, however, they were observed on larger vessels up to 200 μm. The segmental dilatations were never stagnant and never constant in size and position. Sometimes they disappeared quickly with normalization of blood pressure. Frequently, however, the length of the sausages increased, with the narrow segments dilating bit by bit until a situation of diffuse dilatation was produced.

Percentage changes in diameter were much more significant in smaller arterioles than in larger ones. This had already been seen during diffuse hypertensive vasodilatation and was noticed by Suzuki [273] in CO_2-induced dilatation. In arterioles under 30 μm, the mean resting diameter was 19.82 μm at the very place where a sausage-like dilatation would arise during hypertension, and 19.76 μm in the segment between two sausages or at the end of a single one.

Table 8. *Individual Results of Arteriolar Diameter Changes During Acute Hypertension*

Exp.	S			N		
	Resting diameter µm	Maximal diameter µm	%	Resting diameter µm	Minimal diameter µm	%
			I			
F 38 A	25	125	+ 400	20	25	+ 25
B	15	60	+ 300	15	20	+ 30
F 39	300	65	+ 116	25	325	+ 30
F 36 A	30	80	+ 167	28	28	0
B	8	40	+ 400	12	18	+ 50
C	14	40	+ 186	14	16	+ 14
D	10	34	+ 240	12	16	+ 33
F 47	30	85	+ 183	35	45	+ 29
F 50 A	275	100	+ 264	40	27.5	− 31
B	275	82.5	+ 200	20	10	− 50
C	25	95	+ 280	25	20	− 20
F 52	15	40	+ 166	15	15	0
F 53 A	15	30	+ 100	15	10	− 30
B	10	30	+ 200	10	10	0
F 58 A	25	50	+ 100	25	15	− 40
B	10	40	+ 300	10	12.5	+ 25
C	20	35	+ 75	15	10	− 33
			II			
F 38	180	315	+ 75	165	150	− 10
F 47	115	245	+ 113	110	90	− 14
F 52	325	65	+ 100	27.5	32.5	+ 18
F 53 A	75	160	+ 113	65	85	+ 31
B	65	135	+ 108	75	70	− 7
F 58 A	75	115	+ 53	60	65	+ 8
B	75	140	+ 87	60	50	− 17

Exp. = experiment numbers; I = vessels up to 30 µm resting diameter; II = vessels above 30 µm resting diameter; S = segments with sausage-like dilatation; N = narrow segment before or after the sausage-like dilatation; % = percentage diameter increase and decrease, respectively; 0% = resting diameter.

Dilatation was as much as the fivefold of resting values, ranging between + 75% and + 400% above normal (0% = resting value). Mean dilatation was 216.29%. Sausage-like dilatation in vessels larger than 30 µm (32.5–180 µm) was less marked, + 92.71% on the average and 113% maximally (minimum + 53%). Changes in the narrow segments on vessels under 30 µm were not always constriction, but more frequently marked dilatation. Minimum diameter values during the first 5 minutes after onset of hypertension ranged

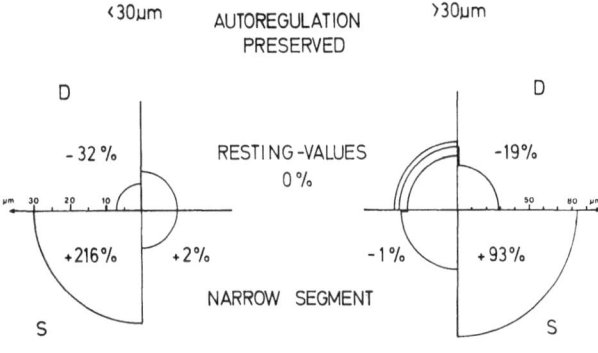

Fig. 29. Comparison of mean vessel diameter changes, showing the occurrences of preserved autoregulation in the upper halves of the graphs. The left graph shows vessels ≤ 30 μm, the right one those > 30 μm. The upper inner quarters show the mean resting diameters of the vessels in absolute and relative (%) terms. Three quartercircles on the right side indicate small differences between the three groups: outer circle = mean diameter before development of sausages; middle circle = resting diameter before diffuse constriction; inner circle = value before formation of narrow segments between sausages. The upper outer quarters give the mean diameters at the moment of maximum diffuse constriction during acute hypertension (D). The lower half of the graph shows diameter changes during breakthrough, when sausages (S) and the narrow segments between them are formed. It may be seen that dilatation in sausage-like deformations is much greater in the small arterioles than in those > 30 μm. Changes in narrow segments average zero in both groups

between — 50% and + 50%, averaging + 1.88%. Arterioles above 30 μm resting diameter changed from — 17% to + 31%, averaging — 1.29%. Resting diameters were 17.5–165 μm, 80.36 μm mean value. They changed to 32.5–150 μm (average 77.50 μm).

Diffuse vasoconstriction occurred at varying times after onset of hypertension and was seen in six out of ten animals without regard to the duration of vasoconstriction and whether it preceded or followed dilatation. Diffuse vasoconstriction was, as mentioned above, the main regulatory mechanism in two of the ten animals, in which constriction persisted until blood pressure had normalized. Thirty-two measurements of different constricted arterioles during hypertension gave the following results: maximal constriction in arterioles under 30 μm resting diameter (7.5–30 μm, mean 18.64 μm) was — 32.09% (— 50 to — 9%), above 30 μm (35–118 μm, mean 67.60 μm) — 19.19% on the average (— 4 to — 40%) (see Table 9). For graphical comparison of different mean diameter changes see Fig. 29. In all groups of animals Evans-blue extravasates were seen

4*

Table 9. *Individual Results of Diffuse Arteriolar Constriction During Acute Hypertension.* For remarks see Table 8

I				II			
Exp.	Resting diameter μm	Minimum diameter μm	— %	Exp.	Resting diameter μm	Minimum diameter μm	— %
F 53 G	12.5	10	— 20	F 53 M	90	87.5	— 4
Q	10	5	— 50	F 52 A	87.5	80	— 9
R	7.5	5	— 33	F 50 A	52.5	42.5	— 19
F 52 E	15	10	— 33	B	50	45	— 10
F	17.5	10	— 43	C	40	35	— 12
F 50 E	20	10	— 50	D	40	27.5	— 31
F 48 H	12.5	7.5	— 40	F 48 A	62.5	55	— 12
F 47 G	27.5	22.5	— 18	B	47.5	40	— 16
K	25	15	— 40	F 47 A	105	90	— 14
F 46 C	27.5	25	— 9	F 39 A	65	40	— 38
F 38 U	30	25	— 17	D	80	75	— 6
				E	60	40	— 33
				F	55	45	— 18
				G	50	30	— 40
				F 38 B	180	150	— 17
				F	40	25	— 37
				G	45	35	— 22
				S	35	25	— 29
				F 36 A	90	75	— 17
				B	85	75	— 12
				C	70	65	— 7

Exp. = experiment numbers; I = vessels up to 30 μm resting diameter; II = vessels above 30 μm resting diameter; % = percentage diameter decrease.

only when vasodilatation had occurred during the hypertensive episode, although the observation of dilatation was not necessarily combined with extravasation.

3.2.7. Discussion

The first observations of pial vessels during acute hypertension date back to a time when the general assumption of cerebrovascular regulation was that of a pressure-passive behavior, resulting in dilatation during hypertension and constriction during hypotension [242], although as early as 1902 Bayliss [30] had found that vessels react to a stretching force with constriction and to a diminution of tension with relaxation. He described this mechanism as "independent of the central nervous system and of myogenic nature".

In 1928 Henry S. Forbes [106] observed that hypertension induced by intravenous injection of epinephrine was followed by pial arteriolar constriction. He concluded from this observation that there apparently must be an active regulatory mechanism governing cerebral vessels. Fog [101] similarly observed this autoregulatory mechanism of vasodilatation with falling and constriction with rising pressure. When Forbes saw dilatation instead of constriction in the "vast majority of cases" in a later study using different concentrations of epinephrine [107], he interpreted the change as distension due to excessive rise in intraluminal pressure. Fog reported the same results in 1938 and saw that "dilatation of the arteries will almost certainly follow if the rise of blood pressure is more than 100%" [101]. I com-

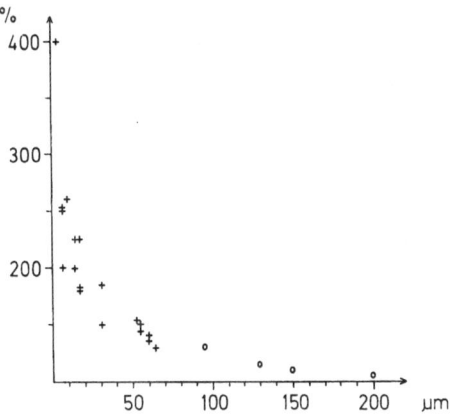

Fig. 30. Some of the first values of percentage arteriolar diameter changes obtained in my own experiments, plotted against resting diameters. ○ = four values as given by Forbes and Wolff coincide nicely with my own results and form a curvilinear relationship

pared my first results with Forbes' measurements, plotting resting diameters against percentage diameter increase and found that both groups of values coincided nicely, forming the typical curvilinear relationship (Fig. 30). The same results were obtained by Riser et al. in 1931 [234] with adrenaline and ephedrine, and by Fog [101—103], who observed "dilatory responses the more often, the higher the pressure increase and the more suddenly it appeared". Thereafter Byrom [55] and Rodda and Denny-Brown [237, 238] observed sausage-string deformation of pial arterioles in chronic experiments and during acute hypertension in chronic hypertension experiments, yet they held the constricted, not the dilated segments, to be pathogenetic. The term "spasm", however, cannot be taken into account on the basis of their experiments, as control pictures of normal pial surface before hypertension and during normocapnia are not available. The results of

Meyer *et al.*, published in 1960 [209], describe arteriolar spasms during acute hypertension. But their figures do also show dilated arterioles ([209]: Fig. 4 B, 10 seconds after onset of hypertension from 110/80 to 250/200) in an example where autoregulation managed to re-establish itself after 30 seconds. Their third figure shows very mild arteriolar constriction during low percentage blood-pressure increase from 120/80 to 165/110. Fig. 7 in that paper [209] also shows transient dilatation of a relatively large arteriole with 136 μm resting diameter which returns to autoregulation after 6 minutes.

Dinsdale *et al.* [68] found dilatation and constriction in the same preparation and thought spasms accounted for the pathological changes, especially spasms after some 8 minutes which were observed following transient dilatation during hypertension. Extravasations of Evans-blue, however, have been observed by others just 20–30 seconds after onset of hypertension [158, 18]. Dinsdale *et al.* did not find any correlation between spasms and degree or duration of hypertension.

Regarding the pathogenetic alterations of pial vessels in acute hypertension, my own results give unequivocal support to the theory that vasodilatation, not constriction, plays the pathological role. The different percentage dilatation of smaller and larger vessels is known from CO_2 reactivity [268, 23, 24] and electrical stimulation [44]. There was no sign of pathologically intensive autoregulation that would be expressed as exaggerated vasoconstriction ending in spasm. Rosenblum *et al.* [239] observed pial vessels in mice during angiotensin-induced hypertension and saw changes similar to those I reported for the animals in group 1. Gannushkina and Shafranova [115] induced acute hypertension in rabbits by intravenous injection of norepinephrine and found dilated segments of pial vessels predominantly in straight anastomotic arterioles in the watershed areas. Hossmann *et al.* [145, 147] obtained similar results during acute hypertension in two different situations, *i.e.*, drug-induced hypertension and after induced tachycardia in cats. Data virtually identical to mine were obtained by the Glasgow group (MacKenzie *et al.* [196], Farrar *et al.* [89], and Strandgaard *et al.* [271]), who completed their work a few months ahead of us. They observed diffuse dilatation in arterioles over 100 μm resting diameter and sausage strings on those below 100 μm, using an image-splitting device. They also described the sausages as a transient phenomenon that frequently changes its shape. Using a method similar to mine, they saw that the narrow segments do not constrict more than they do in the normal autoregulatory range; spasms were never seen. Interestingly, these authors observed increasing rCBF even before arteriolar diameter changes were seen. This result agrees with my own data showing venular dilatation and reddening as the first signs of steeply rising blood pressure. There are, however, some differences between our results, since the experimental approach was somewhat different. The authors used stepwise increase of blood pressure, induced by Hypertensin® and Aramine®; each step was of about 20 mm Hg. Furthermore, they used an open cranial-window technique and described the possibility of ischemic lesions on the preparations due to cerebral edema and herniation. Also, their results were obtained during a period of 90–180 minutes, whereas my observations were made over a period of 5 minutes. They also state that stepwise pressure increase leads to the same results as an abrupt increase, an assumption that is in some contradiction to the results of Häggendal and Johansson, who found cerebrovascular changes only during abruptly induced, but not during stepwise-induced hypertension. It seems possible that small degrees of blood-pressure increase also interfere with autoregulation when the open cranial-window technique is used over a long period and the situation of the intracranial compartments and pressure is altered due to the open bone defect. In addition, it seems unlikely that there is an absolute blood-pressure value of 160–180 mmHg, beyond which cerebro-vascular autoregulation is disturbed in every animal and vasodilatation occurs. It seems more probable that this level, called the "upper limit of autoregulation" is a momentary physiological condition modulated by factors influencing vascular tone such as the level of extracellular bicarbonate, e.g., hydrogen ions, other ions or the sympathicus. That hypocapnia—as performed in my experiments—did not yet afford this protection is not an argument against the assumption of extravascular bicarbonate to be a strong regulating force. Wahl et al. [281] have clearly shown the constrictive effect of sodium bicarbonate, injected into the subarachnoid space immediately adjacent to pial arterioles with a micropuncture technique. My results rather suggest the assumption that the P_aCO_2 was still too high to be able to lower extracellular bicarbonate to an effective degree after the short period of hypercapnia. That hypocapnia, known to cause a decrease in extravascular bicarbonate concentration, offers protection against a breakthrough, has been observed by some investigators[161, 83]. Hypocapnia might, however, have a lesser protective effect than sympathetic stimulation. In addition, an interference between both influential factors, i.e., perivascular hydrogen-ion concentration and the sympathetic nerve, has been reported in both human and animal experiment [62, 79, 144]. This interference decreases the constrictive effect of hypocapnia during sympathetic blockade and the dilatational effect of hypercapnia during sympathetic stimulation [131, 153, 177].

But my experiments do not allow more than an assumption, as perivascular pH was not measured, and there is no information on the real effect of short-term hypocapnia. The same fact must be considered in the experiments involving metabolic alkalosis. Since alkalosis was applied for a longer period of time before the beginning of hypertension, a resulting protective effect is supported by the work of Pannier et al. [225, 224], who demonstrated that blood pH influences CSF pH as a function of time. Thus, CBF decreased after metabolic alkalosis lasting more than 60 minutes. Acute changes in blood pH were, however, ineffective, as other authors have observed [129], [130], [186], [181]; in one series, acute metabolic alkalosis even produced an increase in CBF [128]. This could explain my results showing a protective effect of metabolic alkalosis of about 60 minutes' duration before induction of hypertension. Heuser and Betz [140] held rapid CBF changes after a decrease in blood pH during spontaneous respiration to be a result of respiratory P_aCO_2 change. This possibility cannot be applied to the present results, as the animals were ventilated and kept at a constant P_aCO_2 level.

I did not see pial vasoconstriction immediately after induction of metabolic alkalosis, as described by Wolff and Lennox [290], except when injections were coupled with transitory blood-pressure increase.

The regulation of pH in the CSF and bicarbonate transport through the BBB are not very well understood. Schwab [252] and Fencl et al. [91] proposed an active-carrier mechanism. Metabolic acidosis per se did not affect CBF [129], nor did it facilitate the occurrence of breakthrough.

The vasodilatory effect of CO_2 on pial vessels was discussed above, and in an earlier chapter. That breakthrough of autoregulation was not easier to obtain during hypercapnia than during normocapnia can be related to the low P_aCO_2 values reached in the animals which did not show significant vascular dilatation. In 1965 Harper [130] found that maximal dilatation occurs between a P_aCO_2 of 70 and 80 mm Hg. Johansson found different degrees of extravasation with normo-, hypo- and hypercapnic animals, but significantly higher (60–70 mm Hg) and lower (15–23 mm Hg) CO_2 values were used [161].

Basically, it may now be said that narrowed vessels are less easily affected than predilated ones [80]. This fact will also be shown to influence the extent of extravasation out of altered vessels. This is also made apparent by the vessel-diameter/wall-thickness ratio: the narrower a vessel is, the thicker and therefore stronger its wall becomes, to counteract sudden increase in intraluminal pressure [167].

The effect of the sympathetic nervous system on reactions of pial vessels during stimulation of the sympathetic chain was first observed by Forbes et al. [107], Chorobski and Penfield [57] and Fog [102]. Their uniform results of constriction during stimulation were repeated in a recent study by Kuschinsky and Wahl [180]. Adrenergic nerve fibers which explain this action of the sympathicus have been found in pial vessels of cats [71, 173] (for further references see [77]) and man [74], and recently in intraparenchymal vessels as well [75, 253]. To my knowledge, pial vessels have never been measured during acute hypertension and sympathetic stimulation. The protective effect of this procedure has been assessed by CBF measurements and will therefore be discussed in the appropriate chapter.

There seems to be good evidence now that a high percentage increase in blood pressure within a very short period of time is necessary to produce a breakthrough of cerebrovascular autoregulation in a healthy normotensive subject, and that dilated vessel segments cause further changes. The absolute values of blood-pressure increase and the steepness of increase necessary to produce breakthrough might, however, be a function of the preexistent blood-pressure level. The percentage pressure increase necessary to produce breakthrough might shift towards lower values during stepwise increase when the blood-pressure curve is steep enough from one step to the next. This could explain the discrepancy between the findings of MacKenzie et al. and Häggendal and Johansson, as these two groups had produced stepwise blood-pressure increases of different steepness. It no longer seems tenable to ascribe the main pathogenetic effect to vasospasm and not to dilatation or over-distension during acute hypertension [271, 89]. It appears more probable that such areas of extreme arteriolar constriction can occur during chronic hypertension, as shown by the experiments with chronic renal hypertension. But there would be no proof that such spasms are pathogenetic in nature. In the same way, flow could be increased in another branch feeding such an area through an interarterial connection as has been described by Schmidt [245—250]. This assumption might even be supported by recent investigations by the Meyer group (Mathew et al. [205], who observed decreased blood flow when increasing the blood pressure in hypertensive patients by 30–50%. Normotensive patients showed unchanged flow during this procedure. These results suggest an increased reactivity of brain vessels to increasing blood pressure—as occurs in other vascular beds during renovascular hypertension [60, 93]—in the autoregulatory range of these patients, which is known to be shifted upward (see chapter on clinical considerations). These results do not, however, support cerebrovascular spasms as the main pathogenetic factor of hypertensive encephalopathy and brain edema.

3.3. Reactions of Pial Veins and Their Possible Significance in the Origin of Extravasations

Venous reddening and dilatation were generally the first signs of pial vascular changes in acute hypertension, parallel with rising blood pressure and preceding marked changes in arteriolar diameters. As for their absolute diameter changes, it can be seen that they are not able to dilate to the same degree as arterial vessels (Table 10). As already shown in arterioles, the diameters of small venules also changed more than larger ones. Thus venules with a resting diameter of 7.5–30 µm (mean 23.199 µm) dilated to 16.5–55 µm (mean 33.55 µm), for a percentage increase of 33–167% (mean 73.7%). Venules above 30 µm resting diameter 32.5–285 µm; mean 77.6 µm) dilated to 40–375 µm (mean 96.15 µm, for a percentage increase of 10–76% (mean 31.74%).

Initially, acceleration of venous flow and marked venous reddening were seen together with increasing venular diameters (maximal dilatation was reached after 30 seconds to 3.5 minutes—mean 2.18 minutes). Segmental caliber changes such as the sausage-string phenomenon on arterioles are never seen in veins.

Together with these signs of increasing flow, a marked dissociation in venous outflow began to develop between different venous branches in most of the animals. In one animal, it was even seen during the first 10 seconds and was made visible by deviation of venous flow from one larger draining vein to the region of other draining veins. Very rapid flow, seen on the Evans-blue angiogram, occurs in small branches of deviated venous outflow. Thus, congestion of venous blood can take place all at once in circumscribed areas which, on the one hand, receive a much greater flow rate through the capillary bed. On the other hand, however, this flow is impeded by an equally or still higher venous outflow through a larger branch

Fig. 9. *a* Fluorescence angiogram of normal cat pial vessels. Black line = 66 µm. Arteriole forms a loop before entering the cortex. *b* Typical intervenous connections of the long type, connecting larger venules which are rather far apart

Fig. 10. Fluorescence angiogram of cat pial vessels. Black line = 66 µm. Laminar flow within venules. *a* network of intervenous connections; *b* venule caliber often diminishes at the point of entrance into a larger branch, as also visible in Figs. 6–8

Fig. 31. Evans-blue staining in the wall of an pial artery 15 minutes after onset of acute hypertension. There is, however, no sign of extravasation

Fig. 32. Perivenular Evans-blue extravasations visible on the surface of a cat brain 6 minutes after beginning of acute hypertension

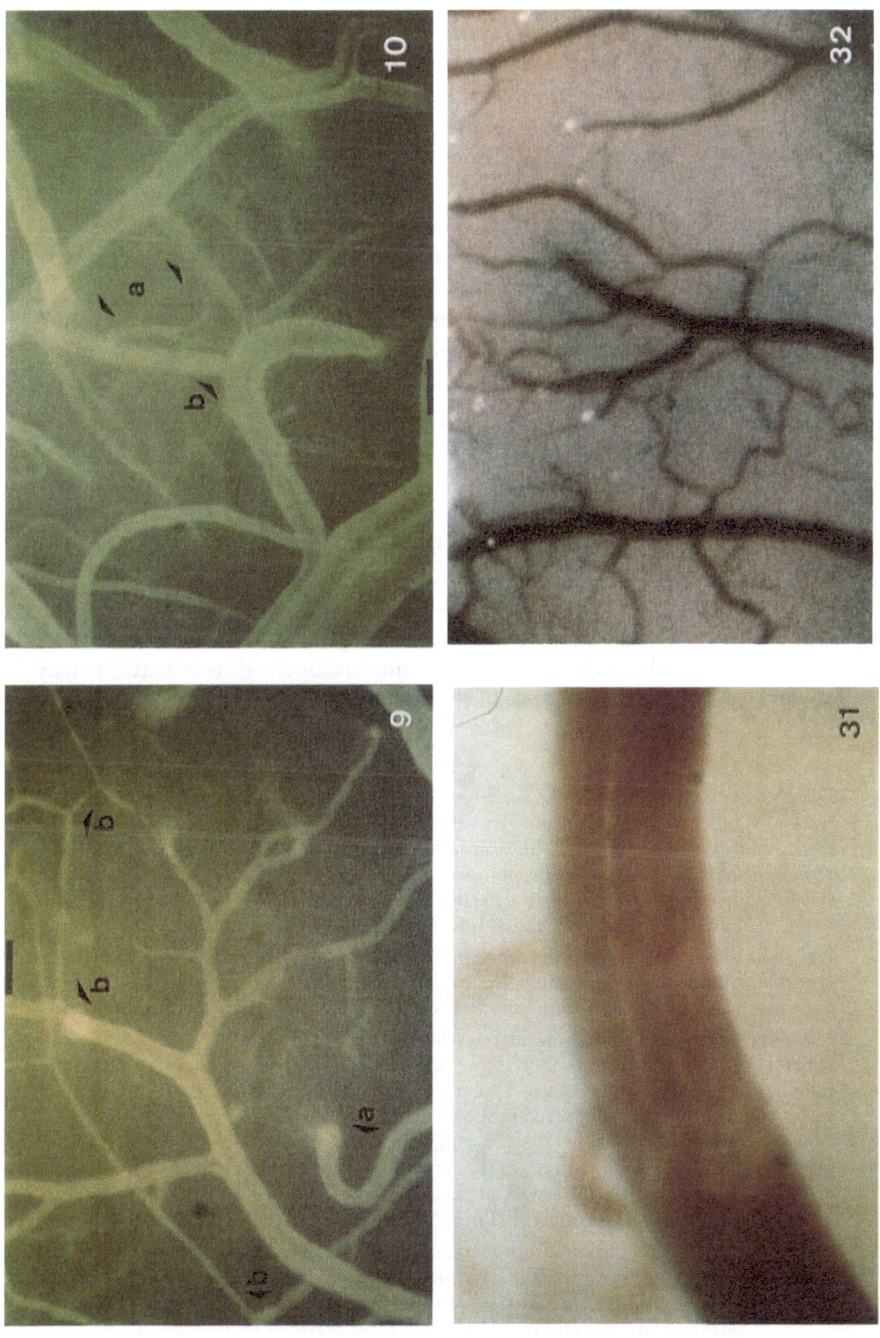

which stops venous outflow in the first. Thus, a situation of insufficiency of venous outflow seems to develop during acute hypertension, although there are many intervenous connections, as previously shown with normal pial vessels. The latter are sometimes dilated during acute hypertension and appear to become a main route of venous outflow from one draining area to another. This, however, is only possible as long as there is a pressure difference between the two outflow areas joined by the veno-venous connection. As soon as flow equalizes on both sides, stasis occurs in these connections, as is frequently seen in the normal situation (Figs. 7 and 8).

The significance of these venular flow characteristics was investigated separately with Evans-blue angiography using the intravital microscope during the first 5 minutes after onset of hypertension, and subsequent photography of a larger brain surface area after 5 minutes through the surgical microscope.

With this routine, Evans-blue extravasation was found only in animals exhibiting diffuse or sausage-like arteriolar changes during hypertension. The development of extravasation was observed in two animals under the glass window in the intravital microscope. In one of them, extravasation could be pursued from the very beginning of hypertension. In other animals patches of extravasate were photographed through the surgical microscope. Extravasation was never seen around arterioles with sausage-like deformation. Only in

Fig. 33. Evans-blue angiography during acute hypertension

Fig. 33 a. Fast flow, stained Evans blue, in the main venous branch (a) 7 seconds after the onset of hypertension. The small venous branches are still red (c). Yet there is a first sign of flow hindrance, because fast-flowing blood in the main branch has already begun to be pumped into the main branch's feeders (d), while the first blue stain is entering the feeder from the capillary bed (e). Fast flow in another venule (f). Black line = 183 μm. MABP = 80 mm Hg

Fig. 33 b. The same angiogram, 1 second later, when blue color has entered the red venous branch (c), indicating the flow direction from postcapillary venules (e) and the main branch (a) into another draining area. Further dilatation of (a).

Fig. 33 c. After 14 seconds, the arteries have turned red, as well as the first small venules with very fast flow (c). Flow in the main branch, however, is severely inhibited, as it still shows dark-blue color and sends blood into the branch (d) which now leads to another draining area (f) via a very short veno-venous shunt (g). The latter is now dilated and also contains blood from a venule with very fast flow (c). Congestion in the main branch now has induced Evans-blue extravasation around the entrances of small branches and around the small branches themselves (h). MABP = 120 mm Hg

Fig. 33 d. Further dilatation of the main branch (a) and stasis in its feeders (d). Expansion of the blue patch (h). The artery, now partly constricting and partly showing sausage-like dilatation (b), shows no sign of extravasation. MABP returned to 120 mm Hg 4.5 minutes after increase to 170 mm Hg

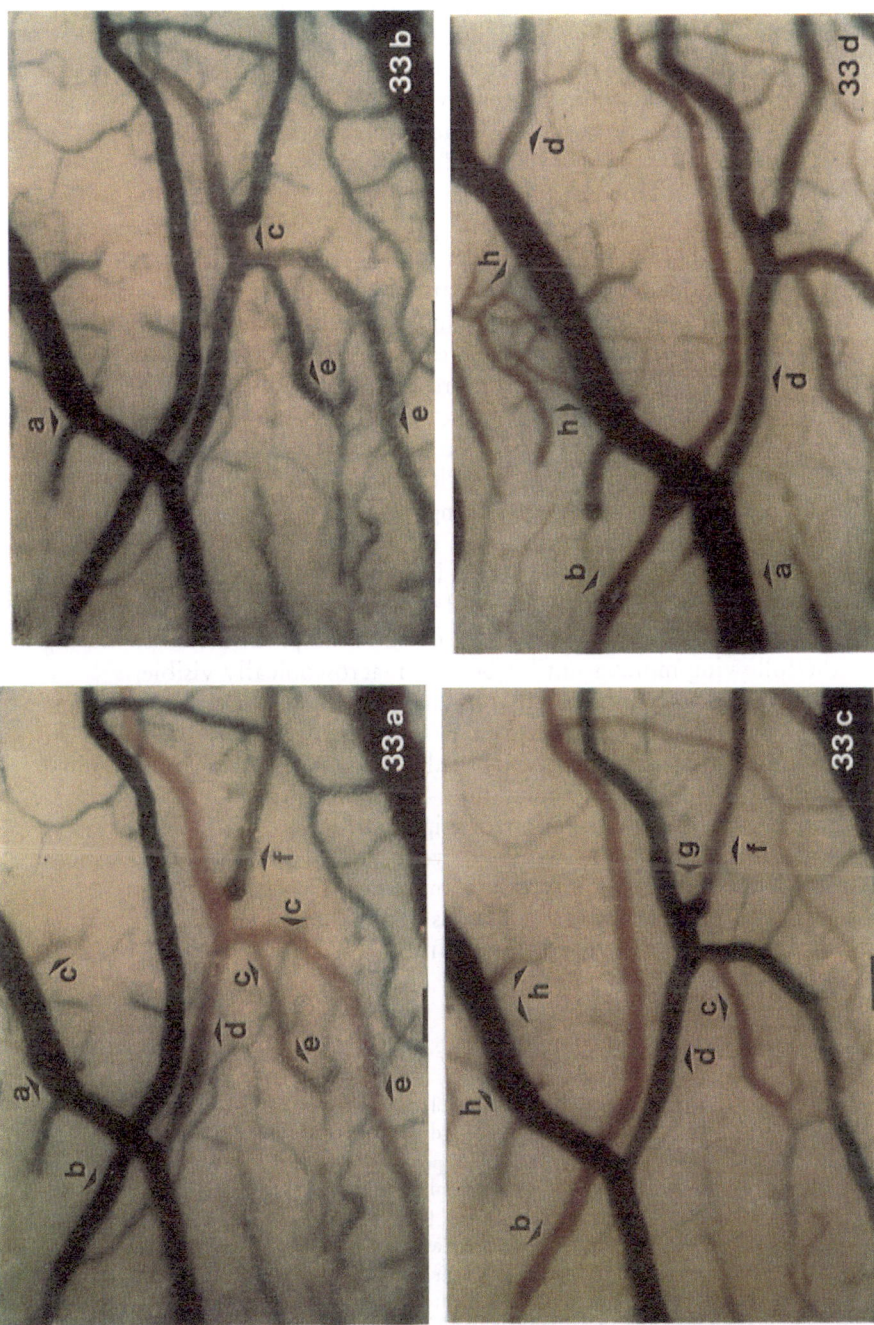

one artery with 198 µm resting diameter could Evans-blue staining
be found in the vessel wall (Fig. 31), exhibiting a uniform consistency.
Small patches were always seen around venules (Fig. 32) or in the
capillary bed, where no extremely dilated arterioles could be found
in the immediate surrounding. The pathogenetic mechanism of extravasation became impressively evident when extremely rapid development of such a blue patch became visible under the intravital microscope (Fig. 33). With rising blood pressure, arteries began to constrict
in the usual way as long as pressure remained within the autoregulatory range. Marked acceleration of venular flow and reddening
of venular blood accompanied this phase and were followed by a
significant dilatation of a venule, while arteriolar sausages developed during further blood-pressure increase. Only 12 to 15 seconds
after the onset of hypertension, the first blue staining was seen around
venules of 20–30 µm entering a larger vein and the major vein itself.
The formation of this patch was clearly related to venous congestion,
visible as long-lasting blue staining, when arterial vessels and other
venules had turned red. Prestasis of small venules and dilatation of
both small venules and the main branch became evident during this
first minute, venular flow being deviated to other main branches via
intervenous connection. The size of the blue patch increased during
the following minutes until it became macroscopically visible.

These results indicate that changes of venous flow during acute
hypertension are more a primary problem of flow speed and its
hindrance than a problem of vascular resistance to high intraluminal
pressure. Changes in venous flow are mainly regulated by increase
in flow speed and deviation of high outflow into regions of lower
outflow through a network of veno-venous connections. Venous
dilatation is not very impressive and seems to be unable—per se—to
eliminate acute elevation of flow, as becomes apparent in the situation
of acute arterial hypertension. Initially, venous outflow becomes

Fig. 34. Multiple, patchy Evans-blue extravasation in a cat-brain cortex 5 minutes
after onset of acute hypertension with blood-pressure increase of more than
100%. Additionally, faint diffuse red-violet staining of astra-violet FF appeared,
indicating the onset of diffuse BBB disturbance

Fig. 35. Evans-blue extravasations occur preferentially in the frontal, parietal and
occipital regions, and generally avoid the temporal lobe

Fig. 36. Under the surgical microscope, blue patches occur around blue-stained
blood vessels, flow together and form a cloudy structure

Fig. 37. Cat-brain section showing an area of Evans-blue staining in the right
anterior caudate nucleus with diffusion into the white matter. This is an extremely
rare observation in all models used in the study of acute hypertension

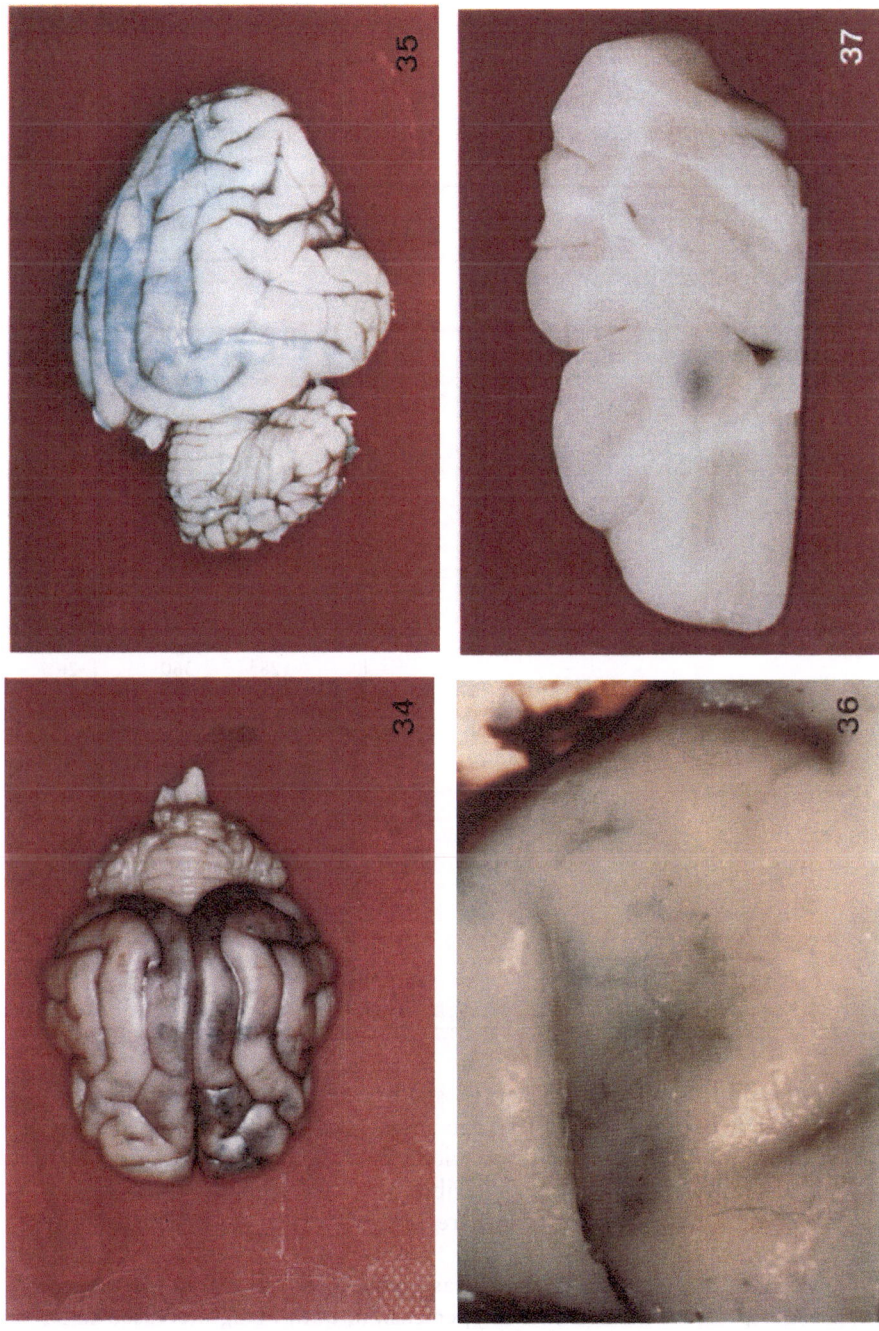

Table 10

Resting diameter up to 30 μm				Resting diameter above 30 μm			
Exp.	Resting diameter μm	Maximal diameter μm	%	Exp.	Resting diameter μm	Maximal diameter μm	%
F 36 G	10.5	16.5	+ 57	F 36 E	54	66	+ 22
N	9.75	16.5	+ 57	F	54	72	+ 33
F 39 Q	30	40	+ 33	F 38 L	45	45	0
F 46 E	27.5	40	+ 45	M	40	55	+ 38
F	30	40	+ 33	N	55	75	+ 36
F 52 N	7.5	20	+ 167	O	60	70	+ 17
F 53 L	25	55	+ 120	P	55	90	+ 64
N	25	42.5	+ 70	F 39 H	75	105	+ 40
O	10	25	+ 150	K	40	65	+ 63
P	25	40	+ 60	L	70	80	+ 14
				M	55	65	+ 18
				N	60	70	+ 17
				O	50	55	+ 10
				P	55	65	+ 18
				F 46 G	47.5	60	+ 26
				L	50	65	+ 30
				F 47 C	100	140	+ 44
				E	285	360	+ 26
				F	235	375	+ 60
				F 48 M	60	70	+ 17
				N	60	82.5	+ 38
				O	35	40	+ 14
				P	32.5	42.5	+ 31
				F 50 G	82.5	145	+ 76
				H	145	210	+ 45
				L	65	105	+ 62
				F 52 G	57.5	70	+ 22
				K	35	45	+ 29
				L	37.5	45	+ 20
				M	32.5	42.5	+ 31
				F 53 K	77.5	95	+ 23

very rapid, subsequently nearly stagnant in a few areas. For the other side of the vascular tree this means that highly increased blood pressure dilates and distends arterioles and capillaries, producing high filtration pressure, but flow is inhibited in some regions where venous congestion takes place, and increases pressure on the arterial and capillary level still further.

These data fit well with measurements of central and cerebral venous pressure during acute hypertension, both being increased to 31 and 27 mm Hg, respectively [124, 125, 123]. They also correlate with pial vessel pressure measurements by Shapiro *et al.* [257]. They found percentage pressure decreases from aortic pressure to larger pial arterioles of 39%, thence to small arterioles around 10 μm of only 10%, and downstream to the veins of another 46%. Stromberg and Fox found the latter measurement to be 40% and wrote that it increased to 52% during hypertension [272]. Together with Häggendal and Johansson's findings [123], these data suggest that the increase in venous pressure during acute hypertension is of great importance, especially in view of the rapid development of extravasation.

The enormously increased amount of blood being pumped through the capillary bed seems to lead promptly to insufficient venous transport, since veins do not dilate to the same extent as arteries. The result is venous congestion in small venules, with an intraluminal pressure somewhat lower than in neighboring ones, so that the blood is prevented from entering a larger vein. Venous congestion in this context has already been considered by Cervos-Navarro [103], who thought it to be caused by compression of bridging veins. Thus, extravasation seems to take place through capillaries and small venules due to highly increased intraluminal and filtration pressure. Evans-blue staining of arteriolar vessel walls can be seen in some instances.

Extravasation, however, was never seen around the arteriolar vessel walls during the acute stage of the type of arterial hypertension described. Suzuki *et al.* observed the pial vessels of cats during acute hypertension using sodium fluorescein as a tracer. They saw extravasations out of all types of vessels [274] but did not comment precisely on the time course of extravasation in relation to pressure increase. The very prompt occurrence of extravasation is, however, not surprising, as Johansson also observed them as little as 30 seconds after the beginning of hypertension [158].

3.4. The Development of Brain Edema

3.4.1. Macroscopy

The occurrence and development of brain edema is a field of preeminent interest as it is known to represent the most severe complication in clinical medicine. Thus Feigin and Popoff [90] and Adachi *et al.* [1] found marked white-matter edema with increased water content in the brains of hypertensive patients. Since the work of B. Johansson, the morphological aspect of protein-rich extravasations due to acute hypertension has become evident [154, 157, 158, 161], when produced either chemically or by clamping of the thoracic aorta.

After staining with the albumin-tracer Evans blue, a patchy pattern of blue staining appears, mainly restricted to the cortical gray matter (Figs. 34 and 35). Special areas on single gyri were preferentially attacked in my experiments, comparable to the watershed zones, as also indicated by other authors [145, 68]. These most peripheral perfusion areas of the three great brain arteries, which coincide and

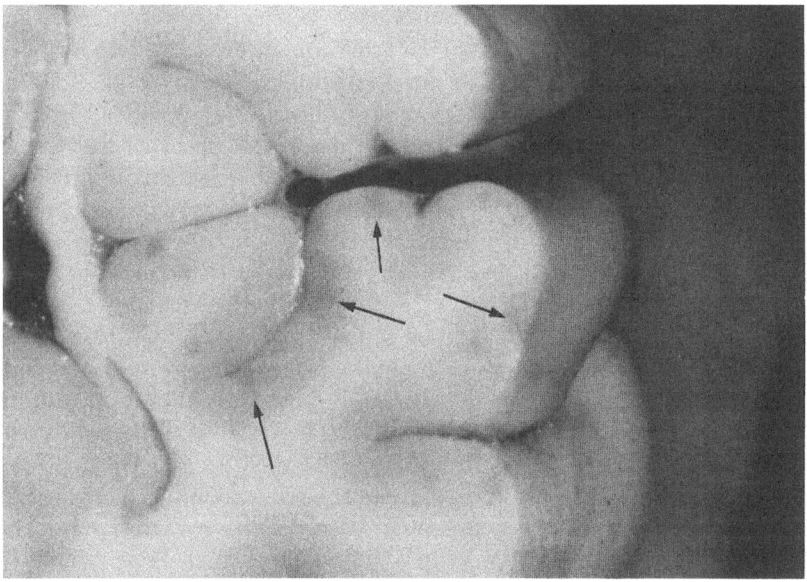

Fig. 38. Coronal cat-brain section showing blue-stained spots restricted to the cortical grey matter

overlap in blood and vascular nerve supply, have been discussed for many years within the context of the pathology of brain circulation [31]. Interestingly, the extent of extravasation correlated very well with the percentage of blood-pressure increase [10], similar to the way arteriolar changes depend on blood-pressure increase. This observation is in accordance with that of Johansson, who saw extravasations only after sudden rise in blood pressure but not after stepwise increase. The results of MacKenzie *et al.* [196], however, showed that breakthrough and extravasation may also occur after stepwise increase, indicating probably the need of a certain steepness of pressure elevation at each step which increases with blood pressure (see also "Pial arterial reactions"). Breakthrough of autoregulation was not necessarily combined with disturbance of the BBB, *e.g.*, not all animals with whatever type of vasodilatation or increased CBF [155, 84] showed Evans-blue extravasations after hypertension. No consistent correlation has yet been found between these two facts.

In brain sections these blue-stained areas turn out to be spherical or cylindrical, sometimes tending to confluence and formation of larger diffuse and cloudy figures which always originate from intensely stained blood vessels (Figs. 36 and 38). In my whole series of experiments I saw only one case with blue staining in the deep structures situated in the caudate nucleus (Fig. 37). White-matter staining, if seen at all, was very faint, in the form of tiny blue streaks, following the direction of the fibers, which turned out to be stained vessel walls. These findings were also confirmed by other investigators [157, 158, 161, 145, 206, 196, 237, 238, 209], although they were ascribed to two different types of pathogenetic mechanisms, as previously mentioned in the discussion of pial arteriolar reactions: Besides distension of the vessel wall by breakthrough of autoregulation followed by BBB leakage, vasoconstriction or vasospasm was given as the cause of these extravasations. My observations of the pial vessels strongly suggest the first theory to explain the morphological changes. The main argument against the vasospasm theory seems, however, to be that extravasations caused by an ischemic lesion would require much more than 5 minutes to become visible [51, 146, 151, 220]. Furthermore, brain energy metabolism turned out not to be disturbed [165]. The localization of these areas with protein extravasation is *not* the same in all types of acute hypertension. Nag et al. [214], using the chemically induced hypertension model in rats, saw trypan-blue extravasations mainly in the temporal cortex and hippocampus. Clamping of the thoracic aorta caused somewhat more frequent extravasations in the basal ganglia than drug-induced hypertension [156]. Spontaneously hypertensive rats were less prone to extravasations during chemically induced hypertension [164]; they were probably protected by the structural changes in the vessel walls. When vessels were predilated by papaverine or hypercapnia, the extravasations were more extensive [124, 157]. Hossmann et al. [147] observed acute hypertension after hypotension during induced cardiac arrhythmia in cats. They did not, however, see any BBB alteration thereafter. An explanation for their failure to observe Evans-blue extravasations in the cortex might be protection of CBF autoregulation by increased sympathetic nerve tone accompanying the spontaneous blood-pressure overshoot which might, in addition, be caused by the sympathetic nerve. A hypertensive crisis provoked by epileptic seizures causes extravasations mainly in the thalamus, rarely in the cortex [166, 227, 190, 193], which is exactly opposed to observations with drug-induced hypertension models. Blue spots were also seen in the cerebral cortex, but they were small and few in comparison to patches in the thalamic region in most animals.

Considering the clinical importance of such extravasation which may be classified as brain edema owing to the elevated tissue water content [55, 237, 238, 209], it would certainly be interesting to know if these blue spots could leak continuously during prolonged hypertension and so account for the origin of severe brain edema. One could imagine a mechanism similar to that observed in the cortical cold-injury experiments, in which edema spread into the white matter [176]. And, in fact, it has been variously demonstrated that white-matter edema exists in the advanced stage of hypertensive encephalopathy'[221]. [1, 209, 55]. An alternative assumption would be diffuse filtration edema. A diffuse BBB alteration may be recognized qualitatively by the observaticn of diffuse staining with astraviolet FF dye [10]. This basic dye enters the endothelial cell as a lipoid-soluble leucobase when hydrogen-ion concentration increases only very slightly and would rather suggest non-vasogenic BBB alteration by tissue acidosis, as may also occur with luxury perfusion [185]. This very sensitive indicator for beginning disturbance of BBB function was first described by Becker and Quadbeck [32, 33] and Gerlach and Becker [117]. When injected intravenously in anesthetized and ventilated control cats, the *in situ* perfused brain (see chapter "Methods") does *not* show any changes. Five minutes after acute hypertension, however, faint diffuse red-violet staining of the cortical grey matter can be seen [10] (Fig. 34). This method is undoubtedly unable to determine the nature of a diffuse type of BBB disturbance in acute hypertension. But it might be a first morphological indicator supporting physiological and morphological data from experiments with hypertension of longer duration [206, 179]. In such experiments, brain water content was seen to be increased in both grey and white matter. One also recalls Byrom's chronic experiments [55]. He described *diffusely* edematous brains after acute hypertensive crisis in renal hypertension.

3.4.2. Fluorescence Microscopy

For fluorescence microscopic observation of the brain in acute hypertension, most of the investigators used Evans blue as a tracer [154, 158, 157, 10]. This substance is known to be bound mainly to albumin [264, 232] when injected intravenously before or immediately after the beginning of hypertension. Extravasation of the dye-protein complex can be found owing to its red fluorescence when longwave ultraviolet light is used as the excitation light in microscopy.

Within just the first 5 minutes after onset of hypertension, vessel-wall staining could be seen on arterioles, capillaries and venules as

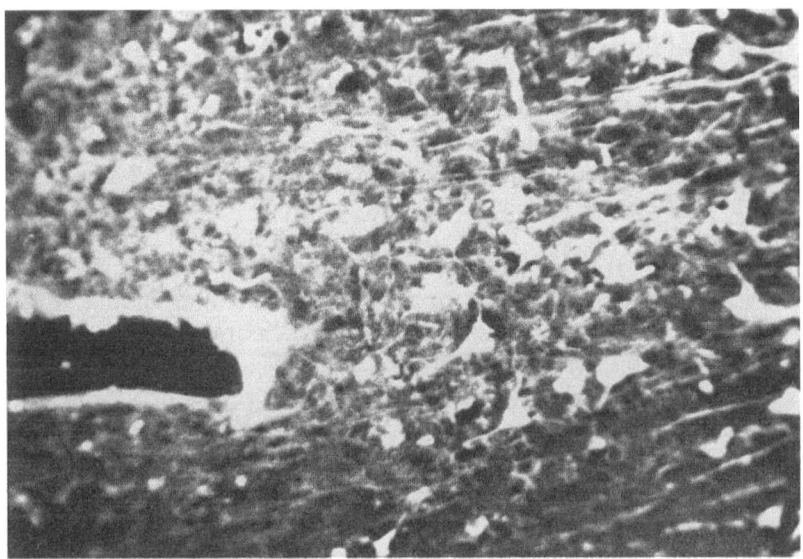

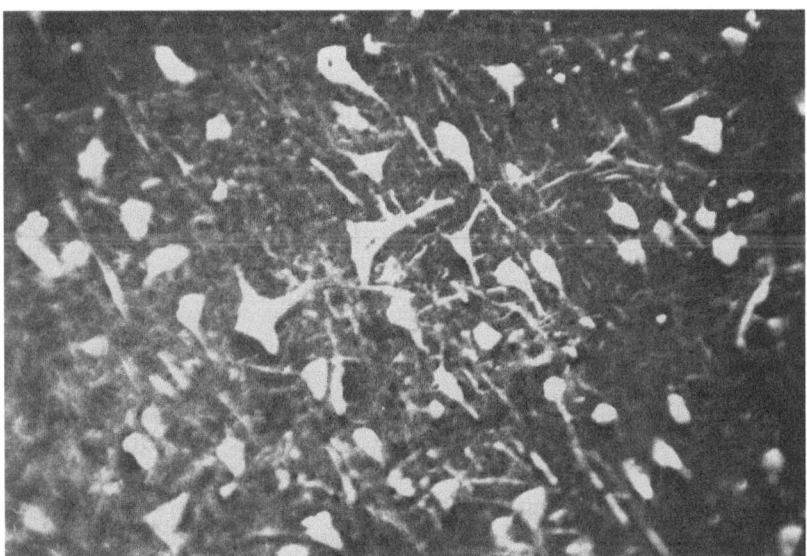

Fig. 39 b

Fig. 39. Evans-blue red fluorescent wall of a cortical venule and diffusely stained neurons and neuronal processes a) in the immediate surroundings and b) remote from the vessel

well as around them. Johansson saw it after 30 seconds on small arteries and arterioles, less frequently on venules. Extravasation was generally described as originating mainly from arterioles [154, 158], although quantitative data are still lacking on this point. Higher magnifications showed the tracer predominantly distributed diffusely in the neuronal cytoplasm and processes, less within the glial cell (Fig. 39). Staining of vessel walls without extravasations can sometimes be observed in areas without pronounced macroscopic blue staining. It was, however, frequently seen within the blue patches, thus giving evidence for the fact that staining of the vessel wall is not necessarily combined with extravasations. This finding also demonstrates that a breakthrough of autoregulation is not always associated with alteration of the BBB; stained vessels may represent distended portions with disturbed autoregulation but with intact BBB. With regard to these histological findings of extravasation as a function of different blood-pressure characteristics, a special type of extravasation after very acute or very high percentage blood-pressure increase was not seen. Red fluorescence was always caused by the same type of extravasate, regardless of size or shape of the blue spots.

3.4.3. Electron Microscopy

Three mechanisms have been discussed as possible origins of extravasation in hypertension: transendothelial vesicular transport, opening of the tight junctions and diffuse passage through the endothelial cells.

3.4.3.1. Transendothelial Vesicular Transport

All authors agree on one observation [214, 179, 88, 119, 126, 284, 287]: endothelial cells within areas of Evans-blue extravasation, and sometimes adjacent areas as well, show a significant increase in the formation of vesicles (Figs. 40 and 41). Following studies with thorotrast and ferritin [263] horseradish peroxidase (HRP) came into common use in recent studies [126, 287, 70, 214] as a protein tracer for ultrastructural study of extravasation mechanisms. The substance has been shown to permeate the BBB under normal conditions in only very small amounts within vesicles [288], but it is capable of demonstrating the greatly increased number of vesicles, filled with reaction product, moving through the endothelium during hypertension. The vesicles begin as membrane invagination on the luminal side and have a diameter of 0.03–0.09 μm. The endothelium is sometimes thickened and may contain a large number of such vesicles forming clusters or

the lumen and ending at the basement membrane. They are often
membrane. The basement membrane is also thickened and of decreased density, sometimes diffuse, sometimes streaky. Another
chains (Fig. 41). These vesicles seem to open towards the basement

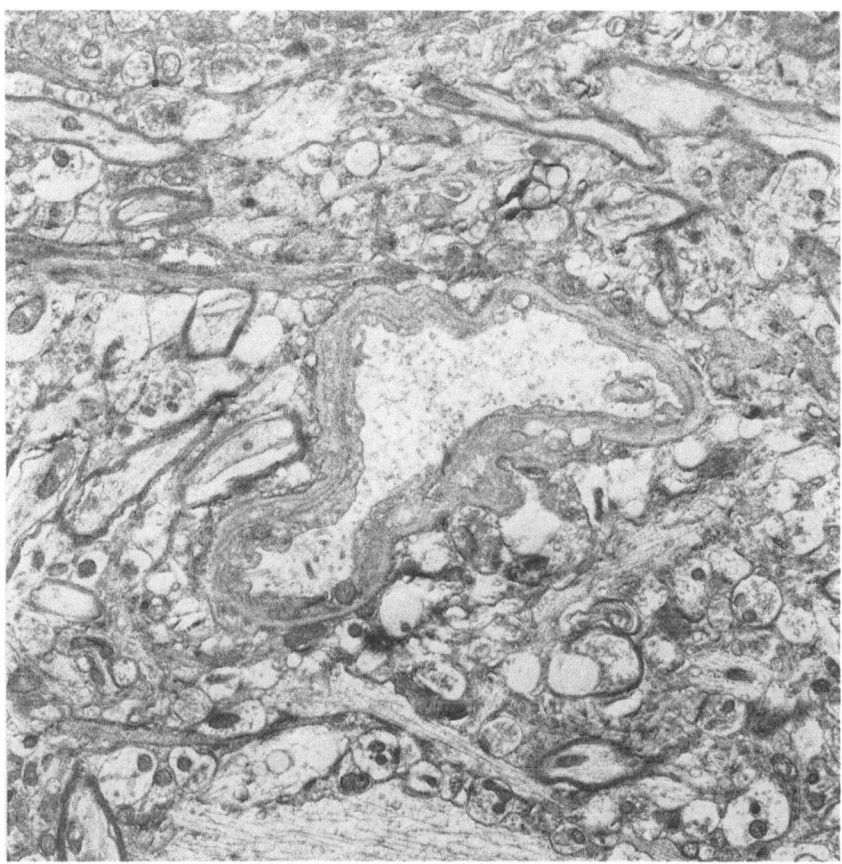

Fig. 40. Electron micrograph of cortical grey matter from an area not stained
with Evans blue 5 minutes after acute hypertension. Magnification ×8,400.
No marked vacuolization of the endothelium, normal structure of the basement
membrane and astrocytic processes

frequent observation is a system of channels or tubules beginning at
curved ("sigmoid shaped", [126]) and difficult to see. On a single section they may appear as vesicles when sectioned transversely. Only
serial sections reveal their real shape, as Hansson et al. demonstrated [126].

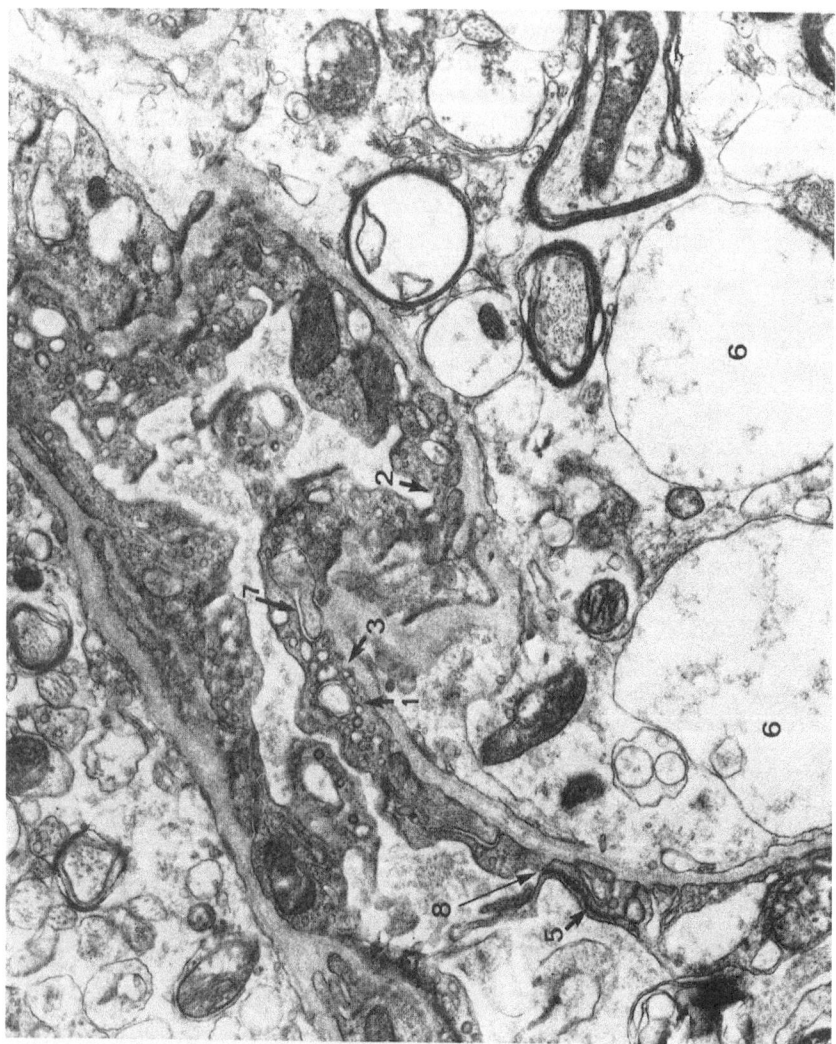

Fig. 41. Electron micrograph of cat cortical grey matter from an area with Evans-
blue staining 5 minutes after beginning of hypertension. *1* Numerous vesicles, in
part forming chains from the luminal side to the basement membrane; *2* invagina-
tions of the luminal membrane; *3* opening of vesicles toward the basement
membrane; *4* thickening of the basement membrane with decreased density;
5 intact tight junctions; *6* swollen astrocytic processes; *7* tubules occasionally
extending from the lumen to the basement membrane; *8* area with very thin
endothelium, and vesicle opening towards the basement membrane

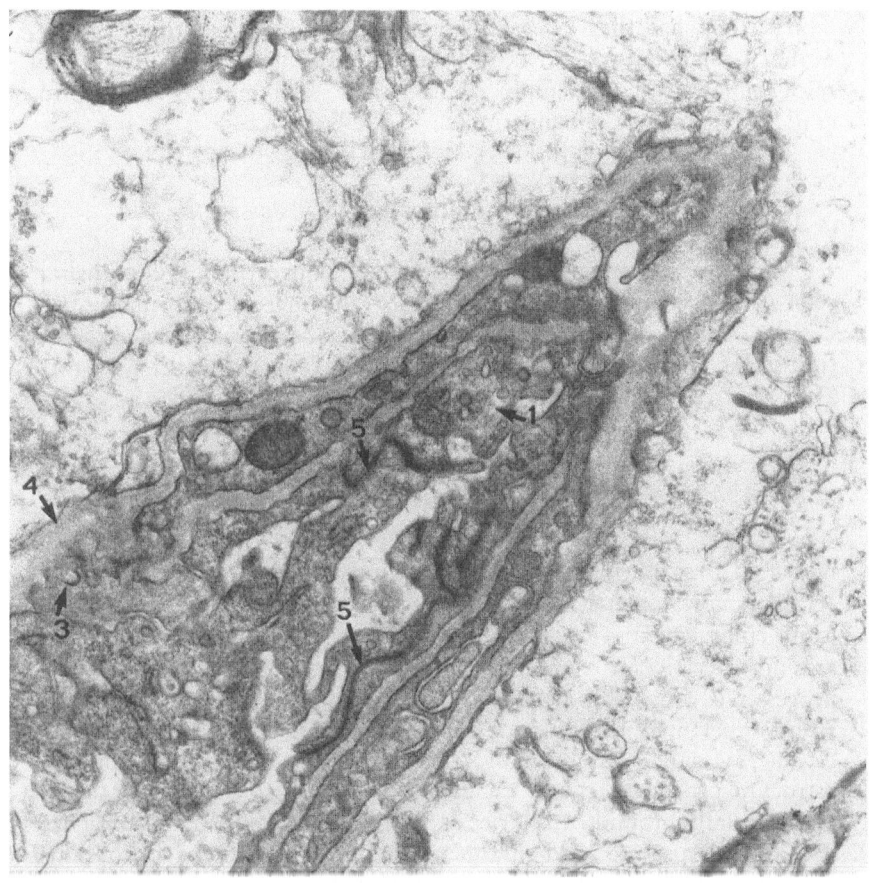

3.4.3.2. Tight Junctions

In all studies on acute hypertension the tight junctions appeared to be normal except in the series of Hansson *et al.* [126], who described occasional observation of HRP reaction product after apparent cleavage of junctional complexes. In a later publication the authors discuss their earlier findings and suggest that the peroxidase seen in a few instances between the endothelial cells could have arrived there by vesicular transport from the adjacent endothelial cells [127]. HRP reaction product was also seen by other authors [214] to fill the junctions from both sides, but to stop at the tight junction itself. The junctions seem, therefore, not to play a primary role as a pathway for extravasation.

In renal-hypertensive rats Giacomelli et al. [119] observed per-oxidase in what they considered to be open tight junctions. These authors suggested that constriction of endothelial cells could be responsible for this opening. In the same experimental model Eto et al. [88] saw intact tight junctions.

3.4.3.3. Diffuse Transendothelial Passage

Most authors stress that there are no changes in the endothelial cells of the cerebral vessels except for the increased formation of vesicles. A diffuse transendothelial passage of tracer substance there-fore seems improbable, although it has been reported to occur in rats after electroconvulsive shock [142].

3.4.3.4. Changes in Astrocytes and Neurons

Astroglial processes are significantly swollen around vessels with increased vesiculation in the endothelium (Fig. 41/6) [214, 284, 70, 88]. In their morphometric study in rats Nag et al. [214] showed a signif-icant enlargement of perivascular processes that was most evident around arterioles. It seems most unlikely that the swelling of astrocyte processes is a fixation artifact, since our own material was obtained from unperfused brains and shows the same results. Westergaard et al. [287] further differentiated this point and reported swelling of astrocyte processes around venules as "an almost constant observa-tion", usually around capillaries as well but not adjacent to arterioles. The authors also reported enlargement of perivascular spaces contain-ing peroxidase and HRP reaction product primarily in the basement membrane of capillaries and venules. Reaction product within glial cells was never seen.

Diffuse neuronal staining with peroxidase—restricted to areas with extravasation—was frequently seen by Nag et al. [214], only seldom by Hansson et al. [126], and never by Westergaard et al. [287]. The mechanisms responsible for these changes are still unclear.

3.4.3.5. Discussion

It is generally agreed that increased transendothelial vesicular transport, apparently triggered by high intraluminal pressure, is the main pathophysiological mechanism leading to protein extravasa-tion [214, 179, 126, 284, 287, 88]. There are, however, some discrepancies in the details. Tubular systems were seen in our material [284] and that of Hansson et al. [126], but not by Nag et al. [214] and Westergaard [287]. With regard to the vessels with the greatest amount of extravasation, our material argues predominantly for capillaries [284]. Hansson et al. saw extravasation in arterioles and capillaries, rarely in venules; Nag et al. generally in arterioles and to an insignificant extent in capillaries and venules. Interestingly, Eto et al. found most marked increases in the number of pinocytotic vesicles in capillaries and venules in renal hypertension. This indicates that we are at present lacking precise data on the quantitatively most important localization of extravasation, although the observation of Westergaard et al. [287] of mainly perivenular astrocyte swelling agrees with my results on pial vessels, seen with Evans-blue angiography. Nag et al. [214] and Olsson and Hossmann [219] observed the direction of vesicular transport when they found tracer in vesicles near the basement membrane 8 and 30 minutes after onset of hypertension, respectively, whereas the luminal side of the endothelium showed vesicles without tracer after 30 minutes.

In some instances the endothelium was very thin in our material and was separated from the basement membrane only by a thin layer of cytoplasm. The vesicles are reminiscent of stomata which recently were reported to have been seen with a scanning electron microscopic technique not only after acute hypertension [132] but also after ischemia [215].

3.4.4. General Considerations on Edema

Cerebral edema is one of the most interesting questions in acute hypertension as it represents an interface of research and clinical work offering the possibility of evaluating experimental data for application in clinical medicine.

Brain edema has been described as a common observation and complication in patients with hypertensive encephalopathy [3, 96, 277, 1, 90, 222]. White-matter edema is usually diffusely distributed and may reach enormous proportions. Now, seeking the origin of hypertensive encephalopathy and observing the patchy pattern of disturbed BBB function, the great challenge arises of determining whether these areas are related to diffuse brain edema and its origin.

Both the morphological and physiological routes have been used to answer the question of the origin of hypertensive encephalopathy and data have been evaluated after different periods of hypertension, thus providing a preliminary concept of the development of edema. Electron-microscopic data [284, 287, 68] have already given us qualita-

tive information on the slight increase in brain volume during the
first 5 minutes of hypertension, when swelling of astrocyte processes
was reported. These findings were supported by a morphometric
study by Nag et al. [213], who found a significant enlargement of
astrocyte processes around vessels within areas of BBB disturbance
when compared to non-permeable areas as soon as 7 minutes after
onset of hypertension. These results per se do not prove the presence
of brain edema, which is defined as increase in tissue water content.
But these results receive physiological support from the chronic
experiments of Byrom [55] and the acute experiments of Meinig
et al. [206], and Meyer et al. [209]. These authors found increased water
content in areas of BBB permeability for protein. These findings are
not basically in conflict with Johansson's negative results [162], as brain
water content measurements had been undertaken on whole rat
brains. During hypercapnic hypertension, water content was also
increased in cortical areas without Evans-blue extravasation [206]. The
extent of brain water increase depended on the duration of hypertension. This observation might be of importance together with
Johansson's [158] results of Evans-blue extravasation which sometimes
continue from the cortex into the white matter. Her results may offer
a connection to data obtained after several hours of hypertension,
which gave evidence of growing diffuse edema, especially in the white
matter. This was first shown by Byrom [55] and later by Kung
et al. [179] and Eto et al. [88].

   This survey of the present state of research allows the hypothesis
to be proposed that cerebral white-matter edema originates in the
cortical areas with BBB disturbance by spreading of the edematous
fluid. More sophisticated and precise methods will be necessary to
test this hypothesis and follow the routes of edema development.

   Our own observation of a diffuse BBB alteration with the astra-
violet-FF dye lacks correlations to other observations, although it
would allow the assumption of a second BBB disturbance during
acute hypertension, diffuse in nature and independent of the circumscribed areas of protein-rich edema. This assumption also bears some
probability, when seen in the light of increasing understanding of the
BBB, which can no longer be viewed as a morphological but rather
as a functional barrier for different groups of substances. Most of
them consume energy and raise the question of brain function and
energy metabolism during acute hypertension, considering the increased transport of substances through the BBB in this situation.
Johansson and Siesjö [165] performed an experiment with rats and
found energy metabolism unchanged. EEG recordings failed to show
major changes besides slight slowing [26, 158, 145].

3.5. Changes in Intracranial and Cerebral Venous Pressure During Acute Hypertension

3.5.1. Intracranial Pressure

Forbes' experiments provided an early description of increase in intracranial pressure during acute arterial hypertension; in these experiments a needle was inserted into the cisterna magna. An insignificant increase in ICP was reported by Byrom [55], who described values in the same range (50–290 mm H_2O) as Forbes. Meyer et al. [209] measured an increase in ICP parallel to blood pressure without giving absolute values. My experiments showed the same percentage increase for ICP as for arterial pressure [11]. Mean arterial pressure increase in a series of six cats was 100%, from 96 to 192 mm Hg. ICP rose from 8.5 to 17 mm Hg. Cerebral perfusion pressure thus could be demonstrated to be enormously increased from 87.5 to 175 mm Hg because the absolute rise in ICP appears unimportant when compared to that of blood pressure. This is a factor of great pathophysiological importance in the pathogenesis of hypertensive encephalopathy. The high discrepancy of the absolute values of CPP and ICP renders most improbable the assumption of the absence of dilatation of capillaries due to the counteraction of increased ICP. It is only in a preexisting pathological situation of increased brain volume or related intracranial masses that ICP begins to play an important role, as it rises more steeply according to another position on the pressure-volume curve when the blood compartment increases in volume [204].

3.5.2. The Venous Volume-Pressure Relationship

ICP and SSSP values are known to be identical in a normal situation, since ICP in the normal situation depends on the intracranial blood volume. The volume of the venous system is dependent on the intravascular pressure. This is illustrative of the passive behavior of these vessels, in contrast to the active autoregulatory mechanism of the arterial vessels. A further contrast to arterial vessels is that venous volume, with pressure rising from zero, does not increase by increasing the vessels' circumference, but by changing its form from a flat structure with collapsed wall first to an elliptic, then to a circular shape, the latter containing the largest volume per unit of vessel length. This volume increase acts as an increase in the blood compartment in the cranial cavity, which leads to a parallel increase in CSF pressure, CSF being the third compartment of the cavity, according to the Monroe-Kelly doctrine, and non-compressible. Up to the point where venous volume increase brings the venous circumferences to a perfectly circular cross-section, venous vessel wall resistance to increasing intraluminal pressure can be held to be practically zero, which means that the intravenous volume-pressure relationship is almost linear up to this point, as shown by Folkow and Neil [106]. Further intravenous pressure increase will lead to further venous dilatation, with intraluminal pressure leading to vessel wall distension. But energy is required to counteract the vessel wall resistance and to reach this vessel volume increase. The volume-pressure relation thus becomes curvilinear, with intravascular pressure increasing more than vessel volume. The higher intraluminal pressure becomes, the more the volume-pressure curve flattens, according to increasing vessel wall resistance, the latter being much higher in venous than in arterial vessels due to their greater content of rigid collagen fibers. The third stage of the volume-pressure relationship in the venous system is represented by the situation of intraluminal pressure at a point where venous wall distensibility has reached a maximum. Here, a further pressure increase will no longer be able to increase venous volume, and the volume-pressure curve becomes horizontal.

Regarding the transmural influence of venous pressure on ICP, changes in the latter will mainly depend on the venous volume-pressure relationship (VVPR), which means that ICP will rise parallel with venous pressure as long as VVPR is linear. Further increase in venous pressure ought to produce a decreasing influence on ICP, until, finally, venous pressure increase no longer increases ICP at all.

3.5.3. The Role of Venous Pressure Increase

Cerebral venous pressure, suggested to equal ICP in acute hypertension, was measured by Häggendal and Johansson [125, 123], who found venous pressure increased up to 17 mm Hg. Superior sagittal sinus pressure was elevated up to 31 mm Hg in their experiments on cats with Aramine®-induced hypertension [124]. These authors concluded that venous pressure increase might play a more important role in the origin of pathomorphological changes than arterial pressure.

Regarding our results in view of the venous volume-pressure relationship, we see that the data follow this relationship exactly. The pressure curves observed during normocapnia would thus reflect a situation in which venous volume begins to increase owing to vessel wall distension, intravascular pressure increasing more than vessel volume. ICP then begins to fall behind venous pressure. During hypercapnic hypertension, total cerebral blood flow is higher than during normocapnic hypertension, as long as hypertension itself does not lead to diffuse maximal vasodilatation. The phenomenon of a breakthrough of cerebrovascular autoregulation with distension of resistance vessels and projection of highly increased intraluminal pressure into the capillary and venous beds occurs diffusely. In this situation of high arterial pressure and vasodilatation it is possible to reach the third stage of the venous volume-pressure relationship, where venous pressure increase is unable to produce further venous volume increase. Here, ICP can remain unchanged with rising SSSP, or decrease during unchanged SSSP.

Simultaneous measurement of intracranial pressure (cisterna magna—ICP), cerebral venous pressure (superior sagittal sinus—SSSP) and arterial pressure (SAP), as described in the "Methods" chapter (see also [316]) showed that ICP and SSSP behave differently. With rising SAP during CO_2-induced vasodilatation, ICP and SSSP increased as well, but SSSP reached higher values, sometimes arriving at the peak value somewhat later than ICP. SSSP remained elevated for a longer time than ICP, thus leading to a further failure of the two curves to run parallel (Fig. 42).

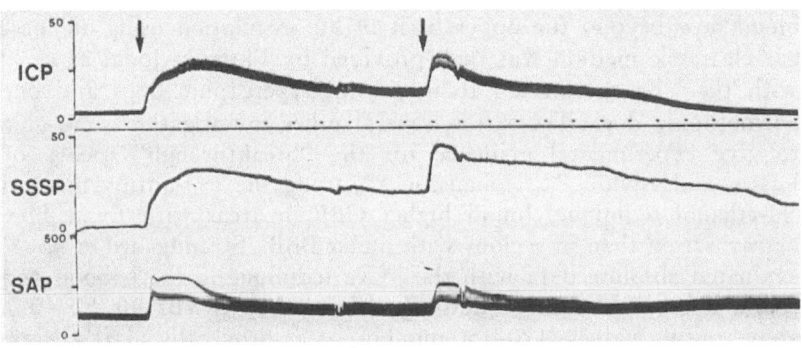

Fig. 42. Simultaneous measurement of arterial pressure (*SAP*) and pressures in the cisterna magna (*ICP*) and superior sagittal sinus (*SSSP*) in a cat during hypercapnia and drug-induced arterial hypertension. Arrows indicate intravenous injection of 200 µg/kg metaraminol (Aramine®). During the first hypertensive episode a P_aCO_2 of 64.5 mm Hg was induced by adding 10% CO_2 to the respiratory gas mixture; during the second episode, CO_2 was increased to 20%, resulting in a P_aCO_2 of 106 mm Hg. It can be seen that SSSP does not parallel ICP, but increases and remains elevated longer than ICP. The markings between the ICP and SSSP curves indicate intervals of 1 minute

Increased venous pressure is thus a plausible factor in extravasation in view of the venous transport capacity, and considering that in my series the relation of mean maximal percentage dilatation of pial arteries and veins during acute arterial hypertension was about 5 : 1 (341% : 74%).

3.6. Cerebral Blood Flow Measurements in Acute Hypertension

The first measurements were performed by Meyer et al. [208] with a thermistor device. They saw initial increase and subsequently marked flow decrease when a thermistor needle was inserted into the cortex. These observations supported the hypothesis that vaso-constriction causes decreased flow and brain ischemia. This remained the main pathogenetic theory of hypertensive encephalopathy for several years. Giese [120], however, observed exudation into the arteriolar wall of mesenteric vessels only in distended vascular portions, an observation which gave a new impetus to the whole field. Byrom [56] reexamined the problem in 1969 and, in the light of Giese's findings and those of Hodge and Dollery on retinal vessels [143], suggested that vasodilatation rather than constriction might be the pathological event. In 1962, Mandel and Sapirstein [201] had pointed out that regional cerebral blood flow, estimated with the [131]J-anti-pyrine technique [243, 244], increased during angiotensin infusion at least by 70%. The first experimental evidence for increased cerebral blood flow beyond the upper limit of autoregulation using an inert gas clearance method was then provided by Ekström-Jodal et al. [83] with the [85]Kr-elimination technique in hypercapnic dogs and one normocapnic dog. Thereafter, several other investigators were able to give experimental evidence for the "breakthrough" theory of Lassen and Agnoli [187]. Johansson [169], using the [125]J-antipyrine and ^{3}H-ethanol technique, found higher CBF in areas with Evans-blue extravasation than in regions with intact BBB. Strandgaard et al. [267] evaluated absolute data with the ^{133}Xe technique in the baboon and found a breakthrough of autoregulation at an MABP of 30–40% above resting values (120–150 mm Hg) as evidenced by marked flow increases (average 50%). The same had been proven by Skinhøj and Strandgaard [260] and Strandgaard et al. [266] one year previously in patients. When repeating these investigations in another series of baboons, Strandgaard et al. [61] reproduced these results. In half of the animals, flow remained elevated after normalization of blood pressure, when the latter was kept above the upper limit of auto-regulation for 10–114 minutes. Analysis of the ^{133}Xe-clearance curves showed that the mean flow increase from 56 to 88 ml/100 g/minute was mainly due to a change of the fast component, while the slow component remained unchanged, thus indicating an increase of grey-matter flow but unchanged white-matter flow. Using the same method of producing acute hypertension by intravenous infusion of angiotensin, Dinsdale et al. [69] measured hyperperfusion during maximum systolic blood pressure, but decreased values thereafter with the ^{14}C-antipyrine method. Focal cortical low-flow areas were maximal after 5 minutes, persisting up to 60 minutes and mainly located in the "watershed areas", the arterial boundary zones. MacKenzie et al. [196] performed CBF measurements using the hydrogen-clearance technique during the experiments cited in the chapter on pial arterial reactions. They also measured marked increase in local flow when pial vasodilatation occurred beyond MABP values of 170 mm Hg. Increases up to more than 250% over the calculated baseline values at 135 mm Hg were seen, although the majority of electrodes had been positioned in the arterial boundary zones. Gannushkina and Shafranova used the same technique and measured values as high as 300% using a further method for assessing CBF, i.e., the labelled microsphere technique [114]. Hossmann et al. [145] induced acute hypertension by intravenous infusion of noradrenaline and measured total flow increase from 33 to 51 ml/100 g/minute, also due to flow increase in the cortical grey matter. Flow was unchanged or even decreased in the white matter, brain stem and cerebellum. In areas with BBB damage, flow rates up to 510 ml/100 g/minute were found.

Despite some basic discrepancies between the different results reported, as cited above, there seems to be enough evidence now that CBF is increased, not decreased, during acutely induced hypertension with whatever method and CBF measured with whichever technique. The observation of highly increased flow in areas of altered BBB permeability to proteins indicates that Evans-blue extravasation does not occur in a situation of vasospasm and ischemia, but of vasodilatation, even distension of the vascular wall. This effect can be damped by stimulation of the cervical sympathetic chain, protracted metabolic alkalosis and hypocapnia [225, 224], and aggravated and supported by hypercapnia [206, 83, 164]. The protective effect of sympathetic stimulation against acute hypertension and breakthrough was established by Bill and Linder [37]. Stimulating one side in cats, they found Evans-blue extravasations and blood-flow increase during acute hypertension mainly on the unstimulated side. Similar results were obtained by Edvinsson et al. in the rat [78]. These findings very much suggest that the sympathetic nervous system (SNS) plays a modulating role in the autoregulation of CBF, stimulation of the SNS shifting the lower and the upper limit toward higher absolute values [200, 172]. Likewise, the lower limit of autoregulation can be lowered by ganglionic blockade [97, 132]. CBF measurements during stimulation in normocapnic animals, where flow reductions of 10% were established, have shown a rather weak influence of the sympathetic nervous system [131, 278] in the normal situation. Decreased

values down to 20% of normal turned out to be technical artifacts [64, 65]. The observation of a greater inhibiting influence of the
sympathetic nerve during hypercapnia than during normocapnia [131]
is a good argument for its modulating character, which tends to
maintain CBF within a normal range; the inhibitory effect becomes
more pronounced with increasing deviation from the normal range.

3.7. General Discussion and Conclusions

3.7.1. Discussion

Acute experiments have been performed in the last few years to
determine the pathogenesis of hypertensive encephalopathy. The
first question arising in this context is, of course, whether acute
experiments can reproduce, physiologically and morphologically, the
situation with which patients present clinically after weeks and
months, or even years. Here, the similarity of several changes seen
in acute and chronic experiments, as mentioned in various chapters,
should be considered. Additionally, seizures were observed in clinical
studies on conscious rats during acute pharmacologically induced
hypertension and chronic renal hypertension [163, 55], although not in
all chronic experiments: 6 of 12 rats with normal resting blood pressure developed generalized convulsions within 1–2 minutes, whereas
10 spontaneously hypertensive animals remained without clinical
symptoms. Studies on the effect of angiotensin—the hypertensive
drug used in this and many other studies—do not suggest such a direct
effect of this substance [256].

Furthermore, it was possible to show that one single short overshoot of blood pressure is able to disturb the cerebrovascular autoregulation of anesthetized animals for a period of time that exceeds
by far that of hypertension [268]. Moreover, the overshoot can also be
responsible for an alteration in the BBB and cause focal extravasation
of serum proteins and water, predominantly into the cerebral cortex.
In this situation pial vessels were distended by highly increased
intraluminal pressure.

Another general question arises when considering the clinical
importance of acute blood-pressure changes, i.e., whether such short
hypertensive phases play any pathogenetic role at all in man. Bevan
et al. [223] showed that blood-pressure values beyond a suggested upper
limit of autoregulation occur in daily life without producing hypertensive encephalopathy. Here, the role of the sympathetic nervous
system must be taken into account as mediator of such hypertensive
episodes that simultaneously increase blood pressure and the upper

limit of cerebrovascular autoregulation, thus preventing breakthrough and brain edema.

Correlating all the different possibilities of pial vascular reactions during different types of blood-pressure increase with the terms "upper limit of autoregulation" and "breakthrough", it becomes difficult to define what may and may not be termed to be autoregulation. It has long been known that rapid blood-pressure changes are, as a first reaction, followed by a pressure-passive flow change. Thus, Fog reported in 1934 that pial arterial vessels took some 90–120 seconds to adapt their diameters to rapid pressure variations [99]. Rapela and Green [230] saw effective autoregulation within 30 to 60 seconds, measuring venous outflow electromagnetically. They considered this autoregulation "most likely to be metabolic of nature". Four years later, Betz reported a time delay of 30 seconds to 2 minutes [36]. Kanzow measured 20–50 seconds [174], Ekström-Jodal et al. 45 seconds as the average of 7 measurements in 4 dogs, the values ranging from 33 to 63 seconds [81]. Symon et al. [275] found an autoregulatory response during pressure increase in baboons of at least as little as 15 seconds, short enough to virtually exclude the possibility that this regulation is metabolic in nature.

Based on this information one might say that arteriolar vaso-constriction after a period of vasodilatation during hypertension can be called "delayed autoregulation", when the constrictive response appears only after several minutes. On the other hand, "delayed breakthrough" may occur when vessels initially constrict and then dilate after some minutes and remain dilated for at least 15 minutes. All these experiments indicate what Ekström-Jodal et al. pointed out in 1971 [83], i.e., that cerebrovascular autoregulation is a "remarkably efficient mechanism" (see also Ekström-Jodal [82]). It is difficult to produce a breakthrough with moderate [291], slow, or stepwise [125] hypertension. Again, very high percentage and steep pressure rise is necessary. That high intraluminal pressure and not another factor causes vasodilatation and focal extravasation was shown by experiments with unilateral carotid ligation [163] to protect the BBB from damage during acute blood-pressure increase. Other arguments have already been given in discussion of the various results in previous chapters.

Considering the lack of correlation between break-through of autoregulation and BBB lesions, several possibilities could be considered. First, it may be assumed that blood pressure must exceed the upper limit of autoregulation by a certain amount before extra-vasation occurs, as CBF begins to increase only beyond this upper limit. This assumption means that a certain excess of CBF rather than a certain blood-pressure level is required to produce extra-vasation, once the upper limit of autoregulation has been exceeded. A wide range of different results becomes possible when the fact is acknowledged that the upper limit of autoregulation is as unknown a factor in every experiment as the resting BP of the animals before induction of anesthesia. Finally, the possibly different effect of the diverse types of anesthesia used in the various studies reported must be taken into account. Sympathetic control turns out to play an important role as "modulator" of CBF regulation. This modulating influence is strong enough to reduce CBF when the sympathetic chain is stimulated during hypercapnia [131, 153, 177]. The reverse, i.e., sympathectomy, would only cause a minimal change in the CO_2 re-activity of brain vessels [265, 285]. Sympathetic stimulation offers effective protection against hypertension by shifting the upper limit towards higher values [37, 40, 100]. On the other hand, vasodilatory agents such as CO_2 [83] or papaverine [157] lower the upper limit, thus facilitating a breakthrough and diffuse vasodistension. It seems most likely that predilated vessels with lower vessel-wall tension are more easily overwhelmed by suddenly rising intraluminal pressure. Two factors might be multiplied, at least during hypercapnic hypertension: the one is the predilatation of vessels, the other their decreased reactivity to sympathomimetic influences due to respiratory acido-sis [282]. This appears to me to be a point of greatest clinical interest, as also noted by Lassen et al. [188]. Giving drugs with vasodilatory action during acute hypertension is no longer recommended, nor should respiratory depressants such as morphines be given, to avoid hyper-capnia and the aggravation of developing encephalopathy [260]. The fact that leakage of proteins occurs more readily in a situation of predilated vessels is a further argument against the spasm theory.

The main transport mechanism of extravasation is transendothelial vesicular transport, described for all types of brain vessels, pre-dominantly arterioles. Venular extravasation seems to result from insufficient venous outflow capacity in regions of greatly increased flow. More precise data on the localization of extravasation and the trigger for enhanced transendothelial vesicular transport are currently under study.

3.7.2. Conclusions

These experiments on the pathogenesis of hypertensive encephalo-pathy and the role of acute hypertensive episodes in the situation of brain injury allow the following conclusions:

1. Cerebral vasodilatation, not constriction, is the pathogenetic

cerebrovascular change causing blood flow alteration and disturbance of the BBB.

2. Narrow segments of vessels in a situation of broken auto-regulation cannot be called spasms.

3. The condition necessary to produce cerebrovascular changes is very steep and high-percentage blood-pressure increase. The percentage of this pressure increase, required to break down autoregulation, was more than 80% in my experiments on normotensive animals. The pressure increase required may diminish with proximity of the "resting" value to the upper limit of autoregulation, if the pressure increase is steep enough.

4. CBF is elevated during acute hypertension, especially in cortical areas with extravasation. White-matter flow remains more or less unchanged during this time. Global flow remains elevated for a certain period after normalization of blood pressure.

5. Vasodilatation and increased CBF are the result of decreased cerebrovascular resistance, overwhelmed by drastically increasing intraluminal pressure.

6. ICP and SSSP increase during acute hypertension is not always parallel. A maximal rise of ICP up to 30 mm Hg is clinically un-important. Venous pressure increase to a still higher degree is able—in this situation of breakthrough and high blood flow—to cause extravasation.

7. Circumscribed areas of serum protein and water extravasation can occur under this circumstance of breakthrough of cerebrovascular autoregulation, but breakthrough is not necessarily accompanied by extravasation.

8. Microscopically, the regions with BBB damage show Evans-blue staining of vessel walls and neurons, increased vesicular transendo-thelial transport, and swelling of astrocyte processes, but normal tight junctions.

4. The Clinical Significance of the Experimental Results

4.1. The Interdependence of Blood Pressure and Intracranial Pressure

H. Cushing [141] first observed that an increase in ICP up to a certain level can result in a concomitant elevation of blood pressure. This event is generally known as the "Cushing reflex" or "Cushing response" and is interpreted as a central regulatory mechanism [286, 183, 178] which maintains adequate cerebral circulation by elevating blood pressure to a certain level above ICP. Johnston et al. demonstrated this effect convincingly [169] with an experiment in baboons: ICP was artificially increased by infusion of fluid into the cisterna magna. At ICP levels between 50 and 100 mm Hg, MABP rose an average of 64%, ranging from 28% to 91% in eight baboons. This hypertension ran parallel with marked increases in CBF (measurement with the xenon-clearance technique), ranging from 26% to 85%. This response of hypertension and high perfusion occurred in all animals except one at ICP levels below that of control MABP and accompanied by failure of autoregulation. With a further increase in ICP, CBF decreased as a linear function of cerebral perfusion pressure. The authors also confirmed an ICP of 50 mm Hg as a critical level, below which CBF remains normal. The occurrence of the Cushing response has recently been considered to depend on sympathico-adrenal discharge at an ICP level around mean or even systolic blood pressure [77]. The reverse situation, *i.e.*, blood-pressure increase during normal resting ICP, would not lead to clinically relevant elevations of ICP, as experimental and clinical data show. This situation is, however, completely altered with brain swelling or other intracranial accumulation of non-compressible material. In this case, the level of ICP becomes more and more dependent on blood pressure [204] and small changes in intracerebral blood volume. The amplitude of pulse-synchronous ICP changes may increase considerably. In such a situation, hypertension might no longer be of importance for the further development of brain edema. Hypertension is, however, increasingly responsible for lowered CPP, leading to a sort of self-restriction of CBF at the level where ICP equals BP. According to the pressure-volume relationship, hypertensive phases aggravate brain edema, especially at the very onset when edema has not yet caused a significant increase in ICP. Thus, CPP becomes enormously elevated and facilitates extravasation through distended vessels, predominantly in regions in which autoregulation had been previously lost.

4.2. Clinical Occurrence of Acute Hypertensive Episodes

The steep and gross blood-pressure increase, experimentally produced with different models such as hypertensive drugs, clamping of the thoracic aorta or of a renal artery, has numerous aspects of clinical relevance. Clinical and experimental observations have shown that epileptic seizures are accompanied by acute hypertension [227, 228, 63, 43]; and, in fact this type of hypertensive episode has been shown to be followed by breakdown of the BBB and extravasations of Evans blue and horseradish peroxidase [63, 42, 43]. Interestingly, these extravasations are not located predominantly in the cortical grey matter, but in the thalamus. Another observation was normal water content in these areas with BBB disturbance. Cerebral blood flow increases by some 100% during seizures, even when normoxia and normocapnia are maintained by artificial ventilation [228, 50].

Other examples of clinical relevance have been found in traumatology. Traumata to the head [8] and spinal cord [122, 61] provoke an acute hypertensive phase very similar to that produced artificially with a hypertensive drug [7, 8, 9]. Griffith [122] reported the occurrence of cortical extravasation of horseradish peroxidase after spinal-cord trauma. Other reports, however, fail to mention cortical extravasation after spinal-cord trauma [61] and after induced tachycardia in cats, followed by acute hypertension [147] (for discussion see chapter "Results"). The aggravating effect of hypertension in situations of disturbed autoregulation and cerebral edema, such as after head injury or brain-tumor surgery, is another relevant clinical observation in this context [203, 13, 14]. This becomes even more apparent from the experimental data presented on acute hypertension. Other experimental data also support this important information: Klatzo et al. [176] induced hypertension after production of a cortical cold injury and significantly higher degrees of brain edema developed in comparison to normotensive animals. In an experimental series in cats, Schutta et al. [251] found marked aggravation of traumatic brain edema when acute hypertension was produced by intravenous injection of norepinephrine.

In the light of present knowledge, the prevention of hypertensive attacks appears to be a significant clinical challenge. These attacks are especially dangerous when normal vessels suddenly become distended due to increasing intraluminal pressure within an injured brain in which circulatory autoregulation has become disrupted. The threat is less apparent in chronic hypertension, in which both the upper and lower limits of autoregulation are known from clinical and experimental work to be elevated [160, 263, 188, 170, 163, 184, 164, 269, 171]. In chronic hypertension vascular resistance appears to become greater owing to structural adaptation [104, 195, 259, 167, 168]. Such patients have normal CBF as long as they do not have cerebral symptoms [184]. The role of cortical low-flow areas in patients with chronic hypertension, as reported by Itoh et al. [152], requires further investigation. The results of these authors from patients with hypertensive stroke lacked evidence of breakthrough during induced mean blood-pressure increase of only 21%.

4.3. Special Reference to Neurosurgical Patients

I may be allowed a few words on the clinical importance of these experimental data for neurosurgery, as I myself am a neurosurgeon. On the one hand, the physiological behavior of the cerebral vasculature can be disturbed by accidental or iatrogenic brain injury. On the other hand, we see vessels with abnormal reactions in and around tumorous tissue. In these situations, an acute hypertensive episode can create considerable problems for both conservative and surgical treatment.

Three typical groups of neurosurgical patients are to be considered: 1. Repeated acute blood-pressure increase in the severely head-injured; 2. intraoperative hypertensive episodes; 3. postoperative hypertensive phases.

Ad 1: Measurements of CBF in head-injured patients may be cited, in which circumscribed areas of highly increased CBF, the so-called "tissue peaks" of washout curves were found [85]. These tissue peaks, indicative of disturbed autoregulation could be provoked by induced hypertension and disappeared during hyperventilation. Furthermore, false autoregulation could be observed especially in patients during the acute stage after severe head injury, when they were comatose and had attacks of decerebrate rigidity [86], apparently when brain edema was most pronounced. This false autoregulation was presumed to derive from passive vasoconstriction caused by edema due to blood-pressure increase and consequent increase in tissue pressure [52, 203, 92]. Based on experimental data on the mechanism of extravasation during acute hypertension, it may easily be imagined how the production of brain edema must be enhanced when blood pressure rises suddenly shortly after trauma.

Table 11. *Evaluation of ICP and SAP in 30 Patients With Severe Head Injuries*
The table shows that a greater percent of hypertensive patients are in the group of nonsurvivors (+) = 69%, whereas 31% of patients with hypertensive blood-pressure values are in the group of survivors (R). Repeated hypertensive crises or persistently high blood pressure can thus be called prognostically bad signs in patients with severe head injury

	R SAP		+ SAP		Total
	> 160 mm Hg	< 160 mm Hg	> 160 mm Hg	< 160 mm Hg	
ICP > 20 mm Hg	5	1	6	2	14
ICP < 20 mm Hg	1	7	7	1	16
Total	6	8	13	3	30

We performed simultaneous measurements of ICP (ventricular catheter) and SAP (radial artery catheter [13], Table 11) in a series of severely head-injured patients and found hypertensive attacks to be indicative of a poor prognosis. These attacks occur mainly as a typical symptom of "acute midbrain syndrome" [118], together with violent phases of extension spasm. They are accompanied by ICP increases (Fig. 43); the degree and amplitude of the increases depend on the enlargement of the non-compressible intracranial compartments, e.g., the extent of brain edema or accumulation of blood or cerebrospinal fluid in the subdural space [138] or cerebral pseudo-tumor [6]. But besides BP-dependent ICP changes, the latter can also increase independent of BP [13].

Regarding the treatment of hypertension in these patients, I should like to stress the importance of simultaneously controlling ICP. It can be dangerous to lower BP when there is no parallel decrease in ICP. When ICP is continuously controlled together with BP, normalization of the latter can, however, allow a quick and effective lowering of excessive ICP [13, 20] (Fig. 44). But the first aim of blood-pressure normalization must be the prevention of excessive brain edema or at least its aggravation [203, 251], and appropriate measures should be taken as soon as possible. In our intensive-care unit, sodium nitroprusside—known as a hypotensive agent for certain neurosurgical procedures—turned out to be one of the most reliable drugs for antihypertensive therapy; its usefulness is, after all, well established in internal medicine (for references see [20]). We have never

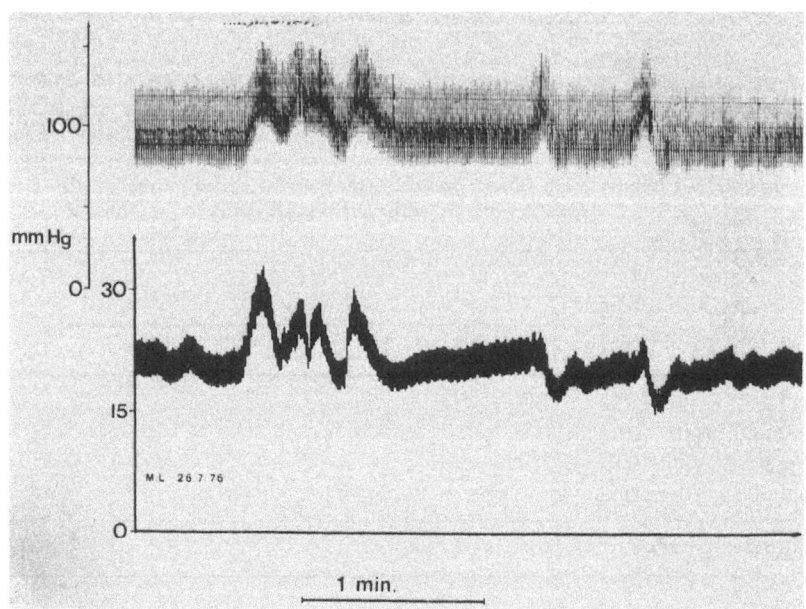

Fig. 43. Arterial pressure (upper curve) and ventricular fluid pressure (lower curve) from a 33-year-old woman after severe blunt head injury. Simultaneous increases in both pressures were recorded during periods of extension spasms in the comatose, assistedly ventilated patient

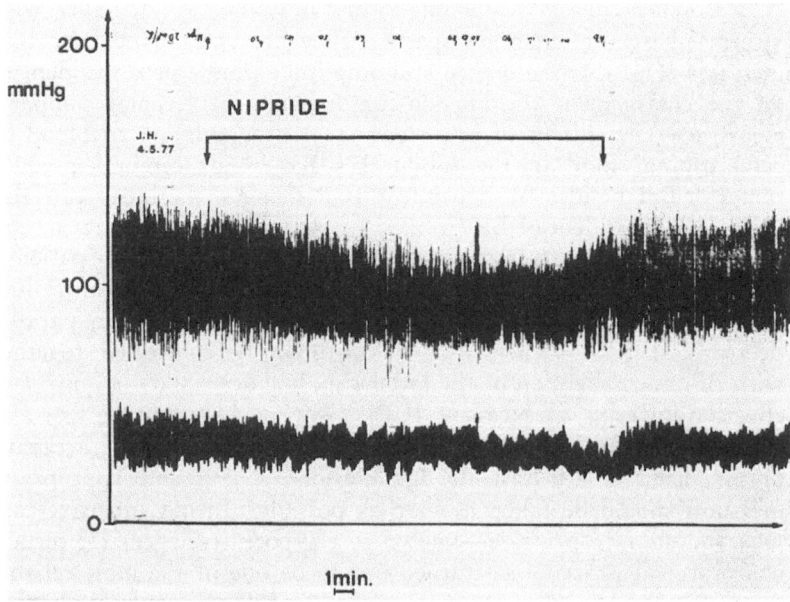

Fig. 44. Upper curve: blood pressure; lower curve: ventricular CSF pressure. Data from a 23-year-old man with severe closed head injury and after evacuation of an epidural hematoma. Parallel lowering of BP and ICP was achieved by intravenous administration of sodium nitroprusside (Nipride). A decrease in ICP amplitude was also attained

seen major complications with this drug and only in very few patients did it fail to lower blood pressure. A great advantage of this drug is that it works very quickly but only briefly; blood pressure may thus be adjusted as desired.

Another attempt to prevent hypertension and its side-effects is the production of an "iatrogenic coma" by barbiturate therapy [202, 87]. These drugs are additionally presumed to act at the molecular level and influence brain metabolic rate [66].

Ad 2: Continuous monitoring of BP during major craniotomies has made us aware of the fact that acute hypertension during surgery frequently causes an inconvenient increase in brain volume which can become a major obstacle during an operation or afterwards, when closing the bone flap may be almost impossible. Therefore we are always prepared to start antihypertensive treatment with sodium nitroprusside [20, 80, 29]. In such cases it may be impossible to lower blood pressure by increasing the dosage of anesthetics, as occurred in the case illustrated in Fig. 45.

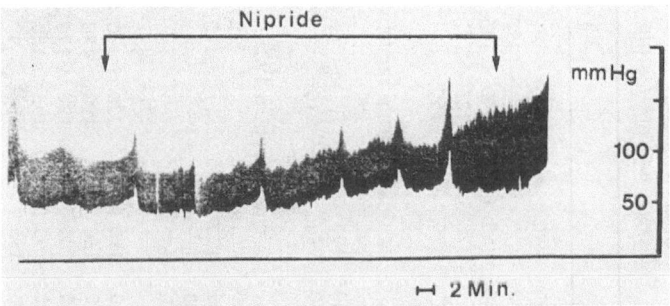

Fig. 45. Blood-pressure curve of a 62-year-old woman during surgery for a pituitary tumor. While the skull was being opened under neuroleptic anesthesia with controlled respiration, systolic pressure suddenly rose to 220 mm Hg. Stepping up the anesthetic dosage did not decrease blood pressure. The hypertensive crisis could be managed only by intravenous administration of sodium nitroprusside (Nipride), beginning with a dosage of 20 ml/hour (1 mg% in 5% glucose solution), which was later increased to 120 ml/hour

Ad 3: Hypertensive episodes in the acute post-operative phase occur mainly within the first 12 hours of intensive care (Table 12). Their combination with minimal clinical symptoms such as headache or drowsiness thus cannot be detected in most cases. Seizures were, however, observed in some instances. Hypertension in this situation might be of some importance for the occurrence of re-

Table 12. Systolic Blood Pressure Values of Patients During the First 7 Hours Postoperative, Given in mm Hg

Age	Diagnosis	0.5	1	1.5	2	2.5	3	3.5	4	4.5	5	5.5	6	6.5	7
66	Meningeoma	170	180				150		190						
63	Metastasis	185		220	160	190		180							
55	Glioblastoma	140	150	130	140	155	170		145		160		150		200
49	Carotid stenosis		170		185		170		next day up to 240	170	200				
61	VIII-Neurinoma		170		150		170	200	190	next day up to 250		190	200	180	170
63	Meningeoma		up to 200 during the first week												
55	Glioma		200		190		200				210	200	200	190	200
59	Carotid stenosis	150	190	150					215						
50	VIII-Neurinoma	230	240		110		140		135		190		100		150
57	Meningeoma	130		140	130			140							
57	Metastasis	195	170	150	140			150		140	120	150		200	
66	Meningeoma		second day up to 190							140			150		
47	Carotid stenosis	200	200							next day up to 240			150		185
53	Meningeoma			180											
62	Glioma	160				135		130		200		180		160	
65	Meningeoma	210	190	210	220	190	210	210	260	120	180	150	175	240	220
63	Meningeoma	140	160	185	190	180	195	180	175	230	160		120	170	165
53	Meningeoma	210	200	180	190	190	190	180	180		180	160	180		100
45	Meningeoma	150	190	210	195	150		150							160
59	Meningeoma	130	185	180	190		190			150		150	160		150
53	Meningeoma	210	200		180		180	170		180	170	160	180		130

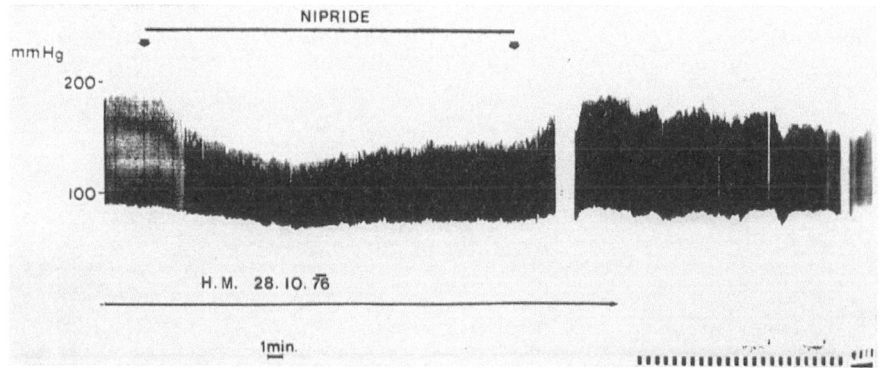

Fig. 46. Treatment of postoperative hypertension. Systolic pressure was lowered from nearly 200 mm Hg to around 130 mm Hg by infusion of 40 ml/hour Nipride solution (50 mg in 500 ml 5⁰/₀ glucose). After treatment, blood pressure remained somewhat below the pretreatment level. Note the decrease in blood-pressure amplitude during normotension

bleeding. The higher frequency of rebleeding in patients with meningeoma might therefore be due to their susceptibility for post-operative hypertension. A small number of patients who had under-gone neurosurgery and their blood-pressure courses are listed in Table 12.

Hypertension aggravates the development of brain edema in brain-surgery patients, just as it does in head-injured patients. Fig. 46 shows the effectiveness of treatment of post-operative hypertension with sodium nitroprusside.

5. Epilogue

The patient reader who has followed me thus far may see, on the basis of these last-mentioned clinical examples, that the experimental work described provided the clinician with valuable pathophysiological and morphological information, and for this reason found immediate clinical application. This material also showed that experimental observations can direct clinical thinking toward a great awareness of the possibly severe consequences of one single symptom, in this case acute hypertension.

Regarding modern intensive-care efforts, present knowledge could challenge us to find a way of artificially maintaining blood pressure at an appropriate mean value in patients with disturbed cerebrovascular autoregulation and blood-pressure dysregulation of whatever origin. This might be the only way to protect these patients from the damaging effect of hypertension, especially acute hypertensive episodes. Automatic blood-pressure regulation might well become one part of an undoubtedly complex system to prevent or limit the development of brain edema. Although the effective treatment of brain edema is still a major problem, especially in acute cases, the possibility of preventing brain edema no longer seems visionary, as studies with preoperative drug treatment have shown [207].

In concluding my survey of recent results on the pathogenesis of hypertensive encephalopathy and the clinical relevance of these data, I should like to request understanding for having possibly underestimated or even omitted the one or the other paper on the subject. The difficulty of writing a scientific monograph including one's own data has always been the overestimation of one's own results. I nonetheless hope to have conveyed the impression that there is general agreement on the essential pathological events leading to hypertensive encephalopathy, and that acute hypertension *per se* can be of considerable clinical importance.

6. Acknowledgements

A major portion of this work was supported by the "Österreichischer Fonds zur Förderung der wissenschaftlichen Forschung".

My special thanks are expressed to Dr. Neuhold for animal care, and to Ch. Adam, K. Wachter, A. Pein, I. Georgiev, and M. Langhart for skillful technical assistance as well as E. Lamont for typing the manuscript.

References

1. Adachi, M., Rosenblum, W. I., Feigin, I., Hypertensive disease and cerebral edema. J. Neurol. Neurosurg. Psychiat. *29* (1966), 451—455.
2. Adler, H., Untersuchungen zur Pathogenese des zerebralen Vasospasmus. Neurochirurgia *17* (1974), 202—208.
3. Alajouanine, Th., Discussion on cerebral edema. Proc. Roy. Soc. Med. *40* (1946), 686—689.
4. Allen, T. H., Orahovats, P. D., Spectrophotometric measurement of the dye T-1824 by extraction with cellophane from both serum and urine of normal dogs. Amer. J. Physiol. *154* (1948), 27—38.
5. Alm, A., Bill, A., The effect of stimulation of the cervical sympathetic chain on retinal oxygen tension and on uveal, retinal and cerebral blood flow in cats. Acta Physiol. Scand. *94* (1973), 84—94.
6. Argyropoulos, G., Der traumatische Pseudotumor des Schläfenlappens und seine Behandlung. Acta Chir. Austriaca, Suppl. *12* (1974), 1—14.
7. Auer, L., Piale Gefäßreaktionen bei akuter Hypertonie — eine intravital-mikroskopische Experimentstudie und deren klinische Relevanz für das traumatische Hirnödem. Wien. Klin. Wschr. *89* (1977), 412—416.
8. Auer, L., Cushing-reflex und Hirnödem. Akt. Traumatologie *6* (1976), 251—255.
9. Auer, L., The role of acute arterial hypertension after head injury. Experimental study in cats. J. Neurosurg. Sci. *20* (1977), 283—288.
10. Auer, L., Brain edema in acute arterial hypertension. I. Acta neuropath. *38* (1977), 67—72.
11. Auer, L., The role of cerebral perfusion pressure as origin of brain edema in acute arterial hypertension. Europ. Neurol. *15* (1977), 153—156.
12. Auer, L., Die normalen Gefäße der Pia mater. Wien. Med. Wschr. In press (1978).
13. Auer, L., Tritthart, H., Ekhart, E., Oberbauer, R., Therapeutic consequences of simultaneous ICP and blood pressure measurement in patients with severe head injury. Proc. 6th Int. Congr. Neurol. Surg., São Paolo, 1977. Exc. Med. *418* (1977), 287.
14. Auer, L., Ascher, P., Tritthart, H., Pathophysiologie des traumatischen Hirnödems. Kongreßbericht Österr. Ges. Chir., pp. 378—381. Graz: Dorrong-Verlag. 1977.
15. Auer, L., Heppner, F., Intravitalmikroskopische Untersuchung der pialen Gefäße. Leitz Wiss. Mitt. In press (1978).
16. Auer, L., A method for continuous monitoring of pial vessel diameter changes. Pflügers Arch. *373* (1978), 195—198.
17. Auer, L., The sausage-string phenomenon in acutely induced hypertension—arguments against the vasospasm theory in the pathogenesis of acute hypertensive encephalopathy. Europ. Neurol. In press (1978).
18. Auer, L., Origin and localization of Evans blue extravasation during acute hypertension. Europ. Neurol. In press (1978).

19. Auer, L., Walter, G. F., Becker, H., Mayer, G., Brain edema in acute arterial hypertension. III. Fluorescence microscopic results. In prep. (1978).
20. Auer, L., Ekhart, E., Bayer, H., The use of sodium nitroprusside as a hypotensive and antihypertensive agent in neurosurgical patients. In prep.
21. Auer, L., Walter, G. F., Reactions of pial vessels to acute arterial hypertension at different levels of arterial pH and carbon dioxide tension. In: Cerebrospinal microcirculation. Ed.: J. Cervos-Navarro. New York: Raven Press. In press (1978).
22. Auer, L., Intravitalmikroskopische Beobachtung der pialen Hirngefäße. Zentralbl. Neurochir. *38* (1977), 175—184.
23. Auer, L., Pial arterial reactions to hyper- and hypocapnia—a dynamic study in cats. Europ. Neurol. In press (1978).
24. Auer, L., Reaktion der pialen Gefäße auf Hypokapnie und Hyperkapnie. In prep.
25. Auer, L., MacKenzie, E. T., Johansson, B., Changes of intracranial pressure and cerebral venous pressure during acute hypertension. In prep.
26. Auer, L., Graham, D., MacGregor, A., MacKenzie, E. T., Johansson, B., Unpublished results.
27. Baez, S., Recording of microvascular dimensions with an image-splitter television microscope. J. Appl. Physiol. *21* (1966), 299—301.
28. Barer, R., A new micrometer microscope. Nature *188* (1960), 398—399.
29. Bayer, H., Auer, L., Ekhart, E., Zur Wirkung von Nitroprussidnatrium bei neurochirurgischen Patienten. In prep.
30. Bayliss, W. M., On the local reactions of the arterial wall to changes of internal pressure. J. Physiol. *28* (1902), 220—231.
31. Becker, H., Die Bedeutung der arteriellen Grenzzonen für die Pathologie der Hirndurchblutung. Dtsch. Zschr. f. Nervenheilk. *164* (1950), 560—568.
32. Becker, H., Quadbeck, G., Tierexperimentelle Untersuchungen über die Funktionsweise der Blut-Hirnschranke. Z. Naturforsch. *7 b* (1952 a), 493—497.
33. Becker, H., Quadbeck, G., Untersuchungen über Funktionsstörungen der Blut-Hirnschranke bei Sauerstoffmangel und Kohlenoxydvergiftung mit dem neuen Schrankenindikator Astraviolett FF. Z. Naturforsch. *7 b* (1952 b), 498—500.
34. Beickert, P., Das Verhalten der Piaarterien nach einseitiger Stellatumblockade und auf einseitigen vegetativen Reiz im Tierversuch. Dtsch. Zschr. f. Nervenheilk. *170* (1953), 285—294.
35. Betz, E., Spontane Schwankungen der Gehirndurchblutung in Narkose und im Wachzustand. Ärztl. Forsch. *21* (1967), 88—89.
36. Betz, E., Autoregulation of cerebral blood flow studied in the brain of cat. In: Blood flow through organs and tissues, p. 257. Eds.: Bain, W. H., Harper, A. M. Edinburgh: Livingstone. 1968.
37. Bill, A., Linder, J., Sympathetic control of cerebral blood flow in acute arterial hypertension. Acta Physiol. Scand. *96* (1976), 114—121.
38. Birch, J., Brånemark, P. I., Nilsson, K., The vascularization of a free full thickness skin graft. III. An infrared thermographic study. Scand. J. Plast. Reconstr. Surg. *3* (1968), 18—22.
39. Birch, J., Brånemark, P. I., Nilsson, K., Lundskog, J., Vascular reactions in a experimental burn studied with infrared thermography and microangiography. Scand. J. Plast. Reconstr. Surg. *2* (1968), 97—103.
40. Boisvert, D. P. J., Jones, J. V., Harper, A. M., Cerebral blood flow autoregulation to acutely increasing blood pressure during sympathetic stimulation. In: Cerebral function, metabolism and circulation, pp. 46—47. Eds.: Ingvar, D. H., Lassen, N. A. Copenhagen: Munksgaard. 1977.

41. Bolwig, T. G., Quistorff, B., *In vivo* concentration of lactate in the brain of conscious rats before and during seizures: new ultra-rapid technique for the freeze-sampling of brain tissue. J. Neurochem. *21* (1973), 1345—1348.
42. Bolwig, T. G., Hertz, M. M., Westergaard, E., The permeability of the rat blood-brain barrier during electrically induced epileptic seizures. Acta physiol. Scand. Suppl. *440* (1976).
43. Bolwig, T. G., Hertz, M. M., Westergaard, E., Blood brain barrier permeability to protein during epileptic seizures in the rat. In: Cerebral function, metabolism and circulation, pp. 226—227. Eds.: Ingvar, D. H., Lassen, N. A. Copenhagen: Munksgaard. 1977.
44. Brandt, H., Enzenross, H. G., The observation of pial arteries—a step to quantify the regulation of the vessels. Drug. Res. *25* (1975), 987—993.
45. Brånemark, P. I., Vitalmikroskopie. Eine Methode für gleichzeitiges mikroskopisches Studium von Struktur und Funktion. Leitz Mitt. Wiss. Techn. *3* (1962), 73—85.
46. Brånemark, P. I., Jonsson, I., Determination of the velocity of the velocity of corpuscules in blood capillaries. A flying spot device. Biorheol. *1* (1963), 143—146.
47. Brånemark, P. I., Experimental biomicroscopy. Bibl. Ant. *5* (1965), 51—55.
48. Brånemark, P. I., Capillary form and function. The microcirculation of granulation tissue. Bibl. Anat. *7* (1965), 9—28.
49. Brånemark, P. I., Intravital microscopy: Its present status and its potentialities. Med. Biol. Illus. *16* (1966), 100—121.
50. Brodersen, P., Paulson, O. B., Bolwig, T. G., Rogon, Z. E., Rafaelson, O. J., Lassen, N. A., Cerebral hyperemia in electrically induced epileptic seizures. Arch. Neurol. *28* (1973), 334—338.
51. Broman, T., The permeability of the cerebrospinal vessels in normal and pathological conditions. Copenhagen: Munksgaard. 1949.
52. Bruce, D. A., Regional blood flow, intracranial pressure and brain metabolism in comatose patients. J. Neurosurg. *38* (1973), 131—144.
53. Bruck, J., Krönke, M., Tschabitscher, H., Arterial hypertension in brain infarction. Incidence, clinical course and angiographic characteristics. In: Cerebral vascular disease, pp. 5—12. Eds.: Meyer, J. S., Lechner, H., Reivich, M. Stuttgart: Thieme. 1976.
54. Bumpus, F. M., Schwarz, H., Page, I. H., Synthesis and pharmacology of the octapeptide angiotonin. Science *125* (1957), 886—887.
55. Byrom, F. B., The pathogenesis of hypertensive encephalopathy and its relation to the malignant phase of hypertension. The Lancet 2 (1954), 201—211.
56. Byrom, F. B., The hypertensive vascular crisis. London: Heinemann monograph. 1969.
57. Chorobski, J., Penfield, W., Cerebral vasodilator nerves and their pathway from the medulla oblongata. Arch. Neurol. Psychiat. *28* (1932), 1257—1289.
58. Clark, E. R., Wentsler, N. E., Pial circulation studied by longcontinued direct inspection. Res. Publ. Ass. Nerv. Ment. Dis. *18* (1938), 218—228.
59. Clark, L. C., Monitor and control of blood oxygen tension and pH during total body perfusion. J. Thoracic Surg. *36* (1958), 488—496.
60. Collis, M. G., Alps, B. J., Vascularreactivity to noradrenaline, potassium chloride and angiotensin II in the rat perfused mesenteric vasculature preparation during development of renal hypertension. Cardiovasc. Res. *9* (1974), 118—126.

61. Collmann, H., Wüllenweber, R., Sprung, Ch., Diusberg, R., Early changes of the spinal cord blood flow regulation in the surrounding area of an experimental injury. In: Cerebrospinal microcirculation. Ed.: Cervos-Navarro, J. New York: Raven Press. 1978. In press.

62. Corbett, J. L., Eidelman, B. H., Debarge, O., Modification of cerebral vasoconstriction with hyperventilation in normal man by thymoxamine. Lancet *11* (1972), 461—463.

63. Cutler, R. W. P., Lorenzo, A. V., Barlow, C. F., Changes in blood brain barrier permeability during pharmacologically induced convulsions. Progr. Brain Res. *29* (1968), 367—378.

64. D'Alecy, L. G., Sympathetic cerebral vasoconstriction blocked by adrenergic alpha receptor antagonists. Stroke *4* (1973), 30—37.

65. D'Alecy, L. G., Feigl, E. O., Sympathetic control of cerebral blood flow in dogs. Circ. Res. *31* (1972), 267—283.

66. Demopoulos, H. B., Flamm, E. S., Seligman, M. L., Jorgensen, E., Ransohoff, J., Antioxidant effects of barbiturates in model membranes undergoing free radical damage. In: Cerebral function, metabolism and circulation, pp. 152—153. Eds.: Ingvar, D. H., Lassen, N. A. Copenhagen: Munksgaard. 1977.

67. Deshmukh, V. D., Harper, A. M., Rowan, J. O., Jennet, W. B., Studies on neurogenic control of the cerebral circulation. Europ. Neurol. *6* (1972), 166—174.

68. Dinsdale, H. B., Robertson, D. M., Chiang, T. Y., Mukherjee, S. K., Hypertensive cerebral microinfarction and cerebrovascular reactivity. Europ. Neurol. *6* (1971), 29—33.

69. Dinsdale, H. B., Robertson, D. M., Haas, R. A., Cerebral blood flow in acute hypertension. Arch. Neurol. *31* (1974), 80—87.

70. Dinsdale, H. B., Robertson, D. M., Nag, S., Haas, R. A., Observation on the nature of blood-brain permeability in experimental hypertension and some effects of horseradish peroxidase. In: Cerebrospinal microcirculation. Ed.: Cervos-Navarro, J. New York: Raven Press. 1978. In press.

71. Donath, T., Monoaminergic innervation of extra- and intracerebral vessels. Acta Morph. Acad. Sci. Hung. *16* (1968), 285—293.

72. Donders, F. C., De bewegingen der hersenen en de veranderingen der vaatvulling de pia mater, ook bij gesloten onnitzetberen schedel regtstreeks onderocht. Onderzoek. Ged. Inh. Physiol. Lab. Utrecht Hoogeoch *2* (1849), 97—128.

73. Dyson, J., Precise measurement by image splitting. J. Opt. Soc. Am. *50* (1960), 754—757.

74. Edvinsson, L., Nielsen, K. C., Owman, Ch., West, K. A., Evidence of vasoconstrictor sympathetic nerves in brain vessels of mice. Neurol. *23* (1973), 73—77.

75. Edvinsson, L., Lindvall, M., Nielsen, K. C., Owman, Ch., Are brain vessels innervated also by central (non-sympathetic) adrenergic neurons? Brain Res. *63* (1973), 496—499.

76. Edvinsson, L., Owman, Ch., Siesjö, B. K., Physiological role of cerebrovascular sympathetic nerves in the autoregulation of cerebral blood flow. Brain Res. *117* (1976), 519—523.

77. Edvinsson, L., MacKenzie, E. T., Amine mechanisms in the cerebral circulation. Pharmac. Rev. *28* (1976), 275—348.

78. Edvinsson, L., Owman, Ch., Pharmacological characterization of adrenergic alpha and beta receptors mediating vasomotor response of cerebral arteries *in vitro*. Circ. Res. *35* (1974), 835—849.

79. Eidelman, B. H., Corbett, J. L., Debarge, O., Frankel, H., Absence of cerebral vasoconstriction with hyperventilation in tetraplegic man. Lancet *11* (1972), 457—460.

80. Ekhart, E., Bayer, H., Auer, L., Nitroprussidnatrium in Neuroanästhesie und Intensivpflege. In prep.

81. Ekström-Jodal, B., Häggendal, E., Nilsson, N. J., Cerebral venous oxygen saturation during rapid changes in the arterial blood pressure. An oxymetric study in dogs. Acta Physiol. Scand. Suppl. *350* (1970), 43—50.

82. Ekström-Jodal, B., On the relation between blood pressure and blood flow in the canine brain with particular regard to the mechanism responsible for cerebral blood flow autoregulation. Acta Physiol. Scand. Suppl. *350* (1970), 1—28.

83. Ekström-Jodal, B., Häggendal, E., Linder, L. E., Nilsson, N. J., Cerebral blood flow at high arterial pressures and different levels of carbon dioxide tension in dogs. Europ. Neurol. *6* (1972), 6—10.

84. Ekström-Jodal, B., Häggendal, E., Johansson, B., Linder, L. E., Nilsson, N. J., Acute arterial hypertension and the blood brain barrier: an experimental study in dogs. In: Cerebral circulation and metabolism, pp. 7—9. Eds.: Langfitt, T. W., McHenry, L. C., Reivich, M., Wollmann, H. Berlin-Heidelberg-New York: Springer. 1975.

85. Enevoldsen, E. M., Cold, G., Jensen, F. T., Malmros, R., Dynamic changes in regional cerebral blood flow, intraventricular pressure, CSF-pH and lactate-levels during the acute phase of head injury. J. Neurosurg. *44* (1976), 191—214.

86. Enevoldsen, E. M., Jensen, F. T., False autoregulation of cerebral blood flow in patients with acute severe head injury. In: Cerebral function, metabolism and circulation, pp. 514—515. Eds.: Ingvar, D. H., Lassen, N. A. Copenhagen: Munksgaard. 1977.

87. Escuret, E., Roquefeuil, B., Frerebeau, Ph., Baldy-Moulinier, M., Effect of hyperventilation associated with administration of central nervous depressants in brain injuries. In: Cerebral function, metabolism and circulation, pp. 154—155. Eds.: Ingvar, D. H., Lassen, N. A. Copenhagen: Munksgaard. 1977.

88. Eto, T., Omae, T., Yamamoto, T., An electron microscope study of hypertensive encephalopathy in the rat with renal hypertension. Arch. Histol. Jap. *33* (1971), 133—143.

89. Farrar, K., Jones, J. V., Graham, D. I., Strandgaard, S., MacKenzie, E. T., Evidence against cerebral vasospasm during acutely induced hypertension. Brain Res. *104* (1976), 176—180.

90. Feigin, I., Popoff, N., Neuropathological changes in late cerebral edema: The relationship to trauma, hypertensive disease and Binswanger's encephalopathy. J. Neuropath. Exp. Neurol. *22* (1963), 500—511.

91. Fencl, V., Miller, T. B., Pappenheimer, J. R., Studies on the respiratory response to disturbances of acid-base balance, with deductions concerning the ionic composition of cerebral interstitial fluid. Amer. J. Physiol. *210* (1966), 459—464.

92. Fieschi, C., Regional cerebral blood flow and intraventricular pressure in acute head injuries. J. Neurol. Neurosurg. Psychiat. *33* (1974), 1378—1388.

93. Finch, L., Häusler, G., Vascular resistance and reactivity in hypertensive rats. Blood vessels *11* (1974), 145—158.

94. Finesinger, J. E., Cerebral circulation I. Arch. Neurol. Psychiat. *28* (1932), 1290—1395.
95. Finesinger, J. E., Cerebral circulation II. Arch. Neurol. Psychiat. *30* (1933), 980—1002.
96. Finnerty, F. A., Hypertensive encephalopathy. Amer. Heart J. *75* (1968), 559—563.
97. Fitch, W., Ferguson, G. G., Sengupta, D., Garibi, J., Autoregulation of cerebral blood flow during controlled hypertension. In: Cerebral circulation and metabolism, pp. 18—20. Eds.: McHenry, L. C., Reivich, M., Wollmann, H. Berlin-Heidelberg-New York: Springer. 1975.
98. Florey, H., Microscopical observations on the circulation of the blood in the cerebral cortex. Brain *48* (1925), 43—64.
99. Fog, M., Om piaarteriernes vasomotoriske reaktioner. Copenhagen: Munksgaard. 1934.
100. Fog, M., Cerebral circulation. The reaction of the pial arteries to a fall in blood pressure. Arch. Neurol. Psychiat. *37* (1937), 351—364.
101. Fog, M., The relationship between the blood pressure and the tonic regulation of the pial arteries. J. Neurol. Psychiat. *1* (1938), 187—197.
102. Fog, M., Cerebral circulation. I. Reaction of pial arteries to epinephrine by direct application and by intravenous injection. Arch. Neurol. Psychiat. *41* (1939), 109—118.
103. Fog, M., Cerebral circulation. II. Reaction of pial arteries to increase in blood pressure. Arch. Neurol. Psychiat. *41* (1939), 260—268.
104. Folkow, B., The hemodynamic consequences of adaptive structural changes of the resistance vessels in hypertension. Clin. Sci. *41* (1971), 1—12.
105. Folkow, B., Neil, E., Circulation, p. 54. London: Oxford Univ. Press. 1971.
106. Forbes, H. S., Wolff, H. G., Cerebral circulation III. The vasomotor control of cerebral vessels. Arch. Neurol. Psychiat. *19* (1928), 1057—1086.
107. Forbes, H. S., Finley, K. H., Nason, G. I., Cerebral circulation XXIV. A. Action of epinephrine on pial vessels. B. Action of pituitary and pitressin on pial vessels. C. Vasomotor response in the pia and the skin. Arch. Neurol. Psychiat. *30* (1933), 957—979.
108. Forbes, H. S., Cerebral circulation XLV. Vasodilatation in the pia following stimulation of the geniculate ganglion. Arch. Neurol. Psychiat. *37* (1937), 776—781.
109. Forbes, H. S., Cerebral circulation XLIV. Vasodilatation in the pia following stimulation of the vagus, aortic and carotid sinus nerves. Arch. Neurol. Psychiat. *37* (1937), 334—350.
110. Forbes, H. S., Vasomotor control of cerebral vessels. Brain *61* (1938), 221—233.
111. Forbes, H. S., Sohler, Th. P., Lothrop, G. N., The pial circulation of normal, nonanesthetized animals. Part 1. J. Pharmacol. Exp. Therap. *71* (1941), 325—330.
112. Forbes, H. S., Study of blood vessels on cortex of living mammalian brain— description of technique. Anat. Rec. *120* (1954), 309—315.
113. Fraser, R., Stein, B. M., Barrett, R. E., Pool, J. L., Noradrenergic mediation of experimental cerebrovascular spasm. Stroke *1* (1970), 356—362.
114. Gannushkina, I. V., Shafranova, V. P., The differences of arterial autoregulation in grey and white matter in acute hypertension, pp. 5.31.—5.35. In: Blood flow and metabolism in the brain. Eds.: Harper, A. M., Jennett, W. B., Miller, J. D., Rowan, J. O. Edinburgh: Churchill Livingstone. 1975.

115. Gannushkina, I. V., Shafranova, V. P., Morphological evidence and pathogenesis concerning the spotty nature of brain tissue damage in experimental hypertensive encephalopathy. In: Cerebral vascular disease, pp. 61—65. Eds.: Meyer, J. S., Lechner, H., Reivich, M. Stuttgart: Thieme. 1976.

116. Gemählich, M., Beitrag zur Technik der intravitalen Auflichtmikroskopie. Z. Wiss. Mikroskopie 64 (1958), 1—12.

117. Gerlach, J., Becker, H., Störungen der Bluthirnschranke bei gedeckten stumpfen Schädelhirntraumen. Z. Naturforsch. 8 (1953), 578—581.

118. Gerstenbrand, F., Das traumatische apallische Syndrom. Wien-New York: Springer. 1967.

119. Giacomelli, F., Wiener, J., Spiro, D., The cellular pathology of experimental hypertension. V. Increased permeability of cerebral arterial vessels. Amer. J. Pathol. 59 (1970), 133—159.

120. Giese, J., Acute hypertensive vascular disease. Acta Path. Microbiol. Scand. 62 (1964), 497—519.

121. Gottschewski, G., Eine neue Methode zur Fluoreszenzmikroskopischen Darstellung der Nierengefäßfunktion im Tierversuch. Ärztl. Forschung 7 (1953), 345—346.

122. Griffith, I. R., Ultrastructural changes in spinal microvasculature after impact injury. Paper given at the International Erwin Riesch Symposium on the Pathology of Cerebrospinal Microcirculation, Berlin, September 7-10, 1977.

123. Häggendal, E., Johansson, B., Pathophysiological aspects of the blood brain barrier change in acute arterial hypertension. Europ. Neurol. 6 (1971), 24—28.

124. Häggendal, E., Johansson, B., Effect of increased intravascular pressure on the blood brain barrier to protein tracers in dogs. Acta Neurol. Scand. 48 (1972), 271—275.

125. Häggendal, E., Johansson, B., On the pathophysiology of the increased cerebrovascular permeability in acute arterial hypertension in cats. Acta Neurol. Scand. 48 (1972), 265—270.

126. Hansson, H. A., Johansson, B., Blomstrand, Ch., Ultrastructural studies on cerebrovascular permeability in acute hypertension. Acta Neuropath. 32 (1975), 187—198.

127. Hansson, H. A., Johansson, B., The cerebrovascular permeability to peroxidase in acute hypertension. A comparison between normotensive and spontaneously hypertensive rats. Acta Neuropath. 1978. In press.

128. Harp, J. R., Gutsche, B. B., Kennell, E. M., Neighy, J. L., Stromberg, E., Wollmann, H., The effect of metabolic alkalosis on cerebral blood flow in man. In: Cerebral circulation and metabolism, pp. 35—37. Eds.: Langfitt, T. W., McHenry, L. C., Reivich, M., Wollmann, H. Berlin-Heidelberg-New York: Springer. 1975.

129. Harper, A. M., Bell, R. A., The effect of metabolic acidosis and alkalosis on the blood flow through the cerebral cortex. J. Neurol. Neurosurg. Psychiat. 26 (1963), 341—344.

130. Harper, A. M., Effect of alterations in the arterial carbon dioxide tension on the blood flow through the cerebral cortex at normal and low arterial blood pressures. J. Neurol. Neurosurg. Psychiat. 28 (1965), 449—452.

131. Harper, A. M., Deshmukh, V. D., Jennett, W. B., The influence of sympathetic nervous activity on cerebral blood flow. Arch. Neurol. 27 (1972), 1—6.

132. Hazama, F., Amano, S., Ozaki, T., Pathological changes of endothelial cells of the cerebral vessels in spontaneously hypertensive rats, with special reference to the role of the cells in the development of hypertensive cerebrovascular lesions. Paper given at the International Erwin Riesch Symposium on the Pathology of Cerebrospinal Microcirculation, Berlin, September 7–10, 1977.

133. Heimberger, H., Beiträge zur Physiologie der menschlichen Kapillaren. Zschr. d. ges. exp. Med. 46 (1925), 519—557.

134. Heine, H., Der Ultropak. Z. Wiss. Mikroskop. 48 (1932), 459—472.

135. Heppner, H., Marx, J. E., Tierexperimentelle Untersuchungen über die Histaminwirkung auf die Endstrombahn des Großhirns. Acta Neurovegetat. 19 (1958), 33—40.

136. Heppner, F., Die Pathophysiologie des sogenannten Gefäßkopfschmerzes. Neurochirurgia 1 (1959), 158—171.

137. Heppner, F., Kapillarmikroskopische Beobachtungen an den Piagefäßen des Großhirns. Acta Neurochir. (Wien) Suppl. 7 (1961), 303—310.

138. Heppner, F., Klinische Neurochirurgie. In: Klinische Chirurgie für die Praxis, Bd. 1, pp. 726—936. Stuttgart: Thieme. 1961.

139. Hernandez-Perez, M. J., Raichle, M. E., Stone, H. L., The role of the peripheral sympathetic nervous system in cerebral blood flow autoregulation. Stroke 6 (1975), 284—292.

140. Heuser, D., Betz, E., Die zeitlichen Änderungen der Gehirndurchblutung bei Alkalose und Acidose des Blutes im akuten Experiment. In: Pharmakologie der lokalen Gehirndurchblutung, pp. 82—87. Eds.: Betz, E., Wüllenweber, R. München: Werk-Verlag Dr. E. Banaschewski. 1969.

141. Heuser, D., Astrup, I., Lassen, N. A., Nilsson, B., Norberg, K., Siesjö, B. K., Are H+ and K+ factors for the adjustment of cerebral blood flow to changes in functional state: "A microelectrode study." In: Cerebral function, metabolism and circulation, pp. 216—217. Eds.: Ingvar, D. H., Lassen, N. A. Copenhagen: Munksgaard. 1977.

142. Hirano, A., Becker, N. H., Zimmermann, H. M., Pathological alterations in the cerebral endothelial cell barrier to peroxidase. Arch. Neurol. 20 (1969), 300—308.

143. Hodge, J. V., Dollery, C. T., Retinal soft exsudates. Quart. J. Med. 33 (1964), 117—131.

144. Hoff, J. T., Sengupta, D., Harper, M., Jennett, B., Effect of alpha-adrenergic blockade on response of cerebral circulation to hypocapnia in the baboon. Lancet 11 (1972), 1337—1339.

145. Hossmann, K. A., Hossmann, V., Tagaki, S., Blood flow and blood brain barrier in acute hypertension. Proc. 8th Salzburg Conference on Cerebral Vascular Disease, 1976. In press.

146. Hossmann, K. A., Olsson, Y., Influence of ischemia on the passage of protein tracers across capillaries in certain blood brain barrier injuries. Acta Neuropath. 18 (1971), 113—125.

147. Hossmann, V., Hossmann, K. A., Hypertensive reaction following induced tachycardia in cats. In: Cerebral vascular disease, pp. 166—170. Eds.: Meyer, J. S., Lochner, H., Reivich, M. Stuttgart: Thieme. 1976.

148. Illig, L., Die terminale Strombahn. Berlin-Göttingen-Heidelberg: Springer. 1961.

149. Intaglietta, M., Tompkins, W. R., Richardson, D. R., Velocity measurements in the microvasculature of the cat omentum by on-line method. Microvascular Research 2 (1970), 462—473.

150. Intaglietta, M., Tompkins, W. R., On-line measurement of microvascular dimensions by television microscopy. J. Appl. Physiol. *32* (1972), 546—551.

151. Ito, U., Go, K. G., Walker, J. T., Spatz, M., Klatzo, I., Experimental cerebral ischemia in mongolian gerbils. III. Acta Neuropath. *34* (1976), 1—6.

152. Itoh, Y., Meyer, J. S., Okamoto, S., Sakaki, S., Miyakawa, Y., Mathew, N. T., Ericsson, A. D., A critical appraisal of the question of "breakthrough" of cerebral autoregulation in patients with hypertensive stroke. In: Cerebral vascular disease, pp. 5—12. Eds.: Meyer, J. S., Lechner, H., Reivich, M. Stuttgart: Thieme. 1976.

153. James, I. M., Millar, R. A., Purves, M. J., Observations on the extrinsic neural control of cerebral blood flow in the baboon. Circ. Res. *25* (1969), 77—93.

154. Johansson, B., Li, C. L., Olsson, Y., Klatzo, I., The effect of acute arterial hypertension on the blood brain barrier to protein tracers. Acta Neuropath. *16* (1970), 117—124.

155. Johansson, B., Strandgaard, S., Lassen, N. A., On the pathogenesis of hypertensive encephalopathy. Circ. Res., Suppl. *1* (1974), 167—174.

156. Johansson, B., Linder, L. E., Blood brain barrier dysfunction in acute arterial hypertension induced by clamping of the thoracic aorta. Acta Neurol. Scand. *50* (1974), 360—365.

157. Johansson, B., Blood-brain barrier dysfunction in acute arterial hypertension after papaverine-induced vasodilatation. Acta Neurol. Scand. *50* (1974 b), 573—580.

158. Johansson, B., Blood-brain barrier dysfunction in acute arterial hypertension. Göteborg: Thesis. 1974 a.

159. Johansson, B., Regional cerebral blood flow in acute experimental hypertension. Acta Neurol. Scand. *50* (1974), 366—372.

160. Johansson, B., Cerebrovascular permeability after angiotensin-induced blood pressure increase in normotensive and spontaneously hypertensive rats. In: Blood flow and metabolism in the brain, pp. 5.3—5.7. Eds.: Harper, A. M., Jennett, W. B., Miller, J. D., Rowan, J. O. Edinburgh: Churchill Livingstone. 1975.

161. Johansson, B., Some factors influencing the damaging effect of acute arterial hypertension on cerebral vessels in rats. Clin. Sci. Molec. Med. *51* (1976), 41—43.

162. Johansson, B., Water content of rat brain in acute arterial hypertension. In: Dynamics of brain edema, pp. 28—31. Eds.: Pappius, H. M., Feindel, W. Berlin-Heidelberg-New York: Springer. 1976.

163. Johansson, B., Hennig, M., The clinical effect of acute blood pressure increase in conscious rats. Acta Physiol. Scand. *98* (1976), 376—378.

164. Johansson, B., Cerebrovascular permeability to protein in spontaneously hypertensive rats after acute blood pressure elevation. Clin. Exp. Pharmacol. Physiol. Suppl. *3* (1976), 97—100.

165. Johansson, B., Siesjö, B. K., Brain energy metabolism in angiotensin-induced acute hypertension in rats. Acta Physiol. Scand. *100* (1977), 182—186.

166. Johansson, B., Nilsson, B., The pathophysiology of the blood brain barrier dysfunction induced by severe hypercapnia and by epileptic brain activity. Acta Neuropath. *38* (1977), 153—158.

167. Johansson, B., Nodborg, C., Cerebral vessels in spontaneously hypertensive rats. In: Cerebrospinal microcirculation. Ed.: Cervos-Navarro, J. New York: Raven Press. 1978. In press.

168. Johansson, B., The cerebrovascular permeability to protein after bicuculline and amphetamine administration in spontaneously hypertensive rats. In prep.

169. Johnston, I. H., Rowan, J. O., Harper, A. M., Jennett, W. B., Raised intracranial pressure and cerebral blood flow. I. J. Neurol. Neurosurg. Psychiat. *35* (1972), 285—296.

170. Jones, J. V., Strandgaard, S., MacKenzie, E. T., Fitch, W., Lawrie, T. D. V., Harper, A. M., Autoregulation of cerebral blood flow in chronic hypertension. In: Blood flow and metabolism in the brain, pp. 5.10.—5.14. Eds.: Harper, A. M., Jennett, W. B., Miller, J. D., Rowan, J. O. Edinburgh: Churchill Livingstone. 1975.

171. Jones, J. V., MacKenzie, E. T., Strandgaard, S., Hypertension and the cerebral circulation. Scot. Med. J. *21* (1976), 103—105.

172. Jones, J. V., Fitch, W., MacKenzie, E. T., Strandgaard, S., Harper, A. M., Lower limit of cerebral blood flow autoregulation in experimental renovascular hypertension in the baboon. Circ. Res. *39* (1976), 555—557.

173. Kajikawa, H., Fluorescence histochemical studies on the distribution of adrenergic nerve fibres to intracranial blood vessels. Arch. Jap. Chir. *37* (1968), 473—482.

174. Kanzow, E., Diskussion zur Pharmakologie der lokalen Gehirndurchblutung. Meßmethoden und Ergebnisse, S. 177—178. Eds.: Betz, E., Wüllenweber, R. Ärztl. Forschg. Suppl. 1969.

175. Klatzo, I., Neuropathological aspects of brain edema. J. Neuropath. Exp. Neurol. *26* (1967), 1—14.

176. Klatzo, I., Wisniewski, H., Steinwall, O., Streicher, E., Dynamics of cold injury edema. In: Brain edema, pp. 554—563. Eds.: Klatzo, I., Seitelberger, F. Wien-New York: Springer. 1967.

177. Kobayashi, S., Waltz, A. G., Rhoton, A. L., Effects of stimulation of cervical sympathetic nerves on cortical blood flow and vascular reactivity. Neurol. *21* (1971), 297—302.

178. Kramer, W., Tuynmann, J. A., Acute intracranial hypertension—an experimental investigation. Brain Res. *6* (1967), 686—705.

179. Kung, P. C., Lee, J. C., Bakay, L., Electron microscopic study of experimental acute hypertensive encephalopathy. Acta Neuropath. *10* (1968), 263—272.

180. Kuschinsky, W., Wahl, M., Alpha-receptor stimulation by endogenous and exogenous norepinephrine and blockade by phentolamine in pial arteries of cats. Circ. Res. *37* (1974), 168—174.

181. Lambertsen, C. J., Semple, S. J. G., Smyth, M. G., Gelfand, R., PH and pCO_2 as chemical factors in respiratory and cerebral circulatory control. J. Appl. Physiol. *16* (1961), 473—484.

182. Landis, E. M., Micro-injection studies of capillary permeability. I. Factors in the production of capillary stasis. J. Amer. Soc. Physiol. *81* (1927), 124—142.

183. Langfitt, T. W., Kassell, N. F., Weinstein, J. D., Cerebral blood flow with intracranial hypertension. Neurol. *15* (1965), 761—773.

184. Lassen, N. A., Cerebral blood flow and oxygen consumption in man. Physiol. Rev. *39* (1959), 183—238.

185. Lassen, N. A., The luxury perfusion syndrome and its possible relation to acute metabolic acidosis localized within the brain. Lancet *1* (1966), 1113—1115.

186. Lassen, N. A., Brain extracellular pH: the main factor controlling cerebral blood flow. Scand. J. Clin. Lab. Invest. *22* (1968), 247—251.

187. Lassen, N. A., Agnoli, A., The upper limit of autoregulation of cerebral blood flow—on the pathogenesis of hypertensive encephalopathy. Scand. J. Clin. Lab. Invest. 30 (1973), 113—116.

188. Lassen, N. A., Strandgaard, S., Skinhøj, E., Cerebral blood flow in patients with arterial hypertension. In: Cerebral vascular disease, pp. 1—4. Eds.: Meyer, J. S., Lechner, H., Reivich, M. Stuttgart: Thieme. 1976.

189. Lebedeva, N. V., The prognostic value of a critical level of arterial blood pressure in patients with hemorrhagic stroke. In: Cerebral vascular disease, pp. 37—40. Eds.: Meyer, J. S., Lechner, H., Reivich, M. Stuttgart: Thieme. 1976.

190. Lee, D. C., Olszewski, J., Increased cerebrovascular permeability after repeated electroshocks. Neurology 11 (1961), 515—519.

191. Leninger-Follert, E., Lübbers, D. W., Interdependence of capillary flow and regional blood flow of the brain. Stroke 4 (1973), 327—328.

192. Leninger-Follert, E., Lübbers, D. W., Wrabetz, W., Regulation of local tissue PO_2 of the brain cortex at different arterial O_2 pressures. Pflügers Arch. 359 (1975), 81—95.

193. Lorenzo, A. V., Shirahige, I., Liang, M., Barlow, C. F., Temporary alteration of cerebrovascular permeability to plasma protein during drug-induced seizures. Amer. J. Physiol. 223 (1972), 268—277.

194. Lübbers, D. W., The oxygen pressure field in the brain and its significance for the normal and critical oxygen supply of the brain. In: Oxygen transport in blood and tissue, pp. 67—92. Eds.: Lübbers, D. W., Luft, U. C., Thews, G., Witzleb, E. New York: Springer. 1968.

195. Lundgren, Y., Hallback, M., Weiss, L., Folkow, B., Rate and extent of adaptive cardiovascular changes in rats during experimental renal hypertension. Acta Physiol. Scand. 91 (1974), 103—115.

196. MacKenzie, E. T., Strandgaard, S., Graham, D. I., Jones, J. V., Harper, A. M., Effects of acutely induced hypertension in cats on pial arteriolar caliber, local cerebral blood flow, and the blood-brain barrier. Circ. Res. 39 (1976), 33—41.

197. MacKenzie, E. T., McCulloch, J., Harper, A. D., Influence of endogenous norepinephrine on cerebral blood flow and metabolism. Amer. J. Physiol. 231 (1976), 489—494.

198. MacKenzie, E. T., McCulloch, J., O'Keane, M., Pickard, J. D., Harper, A. M., Cerebral circulation and norepinephrine: relevance of the blood-brain barrier. Amer. J. Physiol. 231 (1976), 483—488.

199. MacKenzie, E. T., The effect of noradrenaline on cerebral blood flow: the role of the bloodbrain barrier. Thesis, Glasgow 1976.

200. MacKenzie, E. T., McGeorge, A. P., Graham, D. I., Fitch, W., Breakthrough of cerebral autoregulation and the sympathetic nervous system. In: Cerebral function, metabolism and circulation, pp. 48—49. Eds.: Ingvar, D. H., Lassen, N. A. Copenhagen: Munksgaard. 1977.

201. Mandel, M. J., Sapirstein, L. A., Effect of angiotensin infusion on regional cerebral blood flow and regional vascular resistance in the rat. Circ. Res. 10 (1962), 807—816.

202. Marshall, L. F., Shapiro, H. M., Barbiturate control of intracranial hypertension in head injury and other conditions: iatrogene coma. In: Cerebral function, metabolism and circulation, pp. 156—157. Eds.: Ingvar, D. H., Lassen, N. A. Copenhagen: Munksgaard. 1977.

203. Marshall, W. J. S., Brain swelling caused by trauma and arterial hypertension. Arch. Neurol. 21 (1969), 545—553.

204. Matakas, F., von Waechter, R., Knüpling, R., Potolicchio, S. J., Increase in cerebral perfusion pressure by arterial hypertension in brain swelling. J. Neurosurg. 42 (1975), 282—289.

205. Mathew, N. T., Hrastnik, F., Meyer, J. S., Itoh, Y., Miyakawa, Y., Ishihara, N., Is the pathogenesis of hypertensive encephalopathy due to angiospasm or breakthrough? Trans. Amer. Neurol. Ass. 100 (1975), 220—222.

206. Meinig, G., Reulen, H. J., Simon, Ch., Hadjidimos, A., Schürmann, K., Cerebrale Vasoparalyse, arterielle Hypertonie und Hirnödem. J. Neurol. 211 (1975), 25—38.

207. Meinig, G., Aulich, A., Wende, S., Reulen, H. J., The effect of dexamethasone and diuretics on peritumoral brain edema: comparative study of tissue water content and computer tomography. In: Dynamics of brain edema, pp. 301—305. Eds.: Pappius, H. M., Feindel, W. Berlin-Heidelberg-New York: Springer. 1976.

208. Meldrum, B. S., Nilsson, B., Cerebral blood flow and metabolic rate early and late in prolonged epileptic seizures induced in rats by bicuculline. Brain 99 (1976), 526—542.

209. Meyer, J. S., Waltz, A. G., Gotoh, F., Pathogenesis of cerebral vasospasm in hypertensive encephalopathy. I. Effects of acute increases in intraluminal blood pressure on pial blood flow. Neurol. 10 (1960), 735—744.

210. Minard, D., The lucite calvarium for direct observation of the brain in monkeys. Anat. Rec. 120 (1954), 317—330.

211. Molnar, L., Effect of neurogenic hypertension on cerebral blood flow. In: Cerebral vascular disease, pp. 5—12. Eds.: Meyer, J. S., Lechner, H., Reivich, M. Stuttgart: Thieme. 1976.

212. Myers, R. R., Intaglietta, M., Brain microvascular hemodynamic responses to induced seizures. Stroke 7 (1976), 83—88.

213. Nag, S., Robertson, D. M., Dinsdale, H. B., Haas, R. A., Determination of cerebral edema by quantitative morphometry. In: Dynamics of brain edema, pp. 32—37. Eds.: Pappius, H. M., Feindel, W. Berlin-Heidelberg-New York: Springer. 1976.

214. Nag, S., Robertson, D. M., Dinsdale, H. B., Cerebral cortical changes in acute experimental hypertension. An ultrastructural study. Lab. Invest. 36 (1977), 150—161.

215. Nelson, E., Kawamura, J., Sunaga, T., Rennels, M. L., Gertz, S. D., Scanning and transmission electron microscopic study on endothelial lesions following ischemia with special attention to ischemic and "normal" branch points. In: Pathology of cerebral microcirculation, pp. 267—273. Ed.: Cervos-Navarro, J. Berlin: Walter de Gruyter. 1974.

216. Nielsen, K. C., Owman, C., Adrenergic innervation of pial arteries related to the circle of Willis in the cat. Brain Res. 6 (1967), 773—776.

217. Oldendorf, W. H., Brain uptake of radiolabeled aminoacids, amines and hexoses after arterial injection. Amer. J. Physiol. 221 (1971), 1629—1639.

218. Olesen, J., The effect of intracarotid epinephrine, norepinephrine and angiotensin on the regional cerebral blood flow in man. Neurol. 22 (1972), 978—987.

219. Olsson, Y., Hossmann, K. A., Fine structural localization of exsudated protein tracers in the brain. Acta Neuropath. 16 (1970), 103—116.

220. Olsson, Y., Crowell, R. M., Klatzo, I., The blood brain barrier to protein tracers in focal cerebral ischemia. Acta Neuropath. 18 (1971), 89—102.

221. Onoyama, K., Omae, T., Leakage of serum proteins in brain tissues in experimentally induced renal hypertension. Acta Neurol. Scand. *49* (1973), 339—344.
222. Oppenheimer, B. S., Fishburg, A. M., Hypertensive encephalopathy. Arch. Int. Med. *41* (1928), 264—278.
223. Pannier, J. L., Weyne, J., Demeester, G., Leusen, I., Influence of changes in the acid-base composition of the ventricular system on cerebral blood flow in cats. Pflügers Arch. *333* (1972), 337—351.
224. Pannier, J. L., Cerebral blood flow measurements with ^{133}Xenon during experimental alkalosis in the cat. Arch. Int. Physiol. Biochim. *82* (1974), 413—415.
225. Pannier, J. L., Demeester, G., Leusen, I., The influence of nonrespiratory alkalosis on cerebral blood flow in cats. Stroke *5* (1974), 324—329.
226. Peters, Th., Apparatur und Technik zur Mikroskopie an lebenden Säugetier-organen *in situ* in gewöhnlichem Licht und Fluoreszenzlicht. Z. Wiss. Mikr. *67* (1955), 348—367.
227. Petito, C. K., Schaefer, J. A., Plum, F., The blood brain barrier in experimental seizures. In: Dynamics of brain edema, pp. 38—42. Eds.: Pappius, H. M., Feindel, W. Berlin-Heidelberg-New York: Springer. 1976.
228. Plum, F., Posner, J., Troy, B., Cerebral metabolism and circulatory response to induced convulsions in animals. Arch. Neurol. *18* (1968), 1—13.
229. Pool, J. L., Cerebral circulation. XXII. Effect of stimulation of the sympathetic nerve on the pial vessels in the isolated head. Arch. Neurol. Psychiat. *32* (1934), 916—923.
230. Rapela, C. E., Green, H. D., Autoregulation of canine cerebral blood flow. Circ. Res. Suppl. *1* (1964), 205—211.
231. Raper, A. J., Kontos, H. A., Patterson, J. L., Response of pial precapillary vessels to changes in arterial carbon dioxide tension. Circ. Res. *28* (1971), 518—523.
232. Rawson, R. A., The binding of T-1824 and structurally related diazo-dyes by the plasma proteins. Amer. J. Physiol. *138* (1943), 708—717.
233. Reid, I. A., Is there a brain renin-angiotensin system? Circ. Res. *41* (1977), 147—153.
234. Riser, M., Meriel, P., Planques, F., Les spasmes vasculaires en neurologie — étude clinique et expérimentale. Encéphale *26* (1931), 501—528.
235. Rittel, W., Iselin, B., Kappeler, H., Riniker, B., Schwyzer, R., Synthese eines hochwirksamen Hypertensin-II-Amids. Helv. Chim. Acta *15* (1957), 614—624.
236. Robertson, D. M., Experimental hypertensive cerebrovascular disease. Amer. J. Pathol. *59* (1969), 63—89.
237. Rodda, R., Denny-Brown, D., The cerebral arterioles in experimental hypertension. I. Amer. J. Pathol. *49* (1966), 53—76.
238. Rodda, R., Denny-Brown, D., The cerebral arterioles in experimental hypertension. Amer. J. Pathol. *49* (1966), 365—381.
239. Rosenblum, W. I., Donnenfeld, H., Aleu, F., Effects of increased blood pressure on cerebral vessels in mice. Arch. Neurol. *14* (1966), 631—643.
240. Rosenblum, W. I., Fluorescence angiography of cerebral microcirculation. Amer. J. Pathol. *59* (1969), 9.
241. Rosenblum, W. I., Effects of blood pressure and blood viscosity on fluorescein transit time in the cerebral microcirculation in the mouse. Circ. Res. *27* (1970), 825—833.
242. Roy, C. S., Sherrington, C. S., On the regulation of the blood supply of the brain. J. Physiol. *17* (1890), 85—108.

243. Sapirstein, L. A., Regional blood flow by fractional distribution of indicators. Amer. J. Physiol. *193* (1958), 161—168.
244. Sapirstein, L. A., Mandel, M. J., Blood flow in the aortic wall. Circ. Res. 7 (1959), 549—560.
245. Schmidt, H. W., Über Arterienkreise in der Pia mater des Menschen. Dtsch. Z. Nervenheilk. *172* (1955), 526—530.
246. Schmidt, H. W., Über Embolien in den Arterienkreisen der Pia mater. Z. Ges. Exp. Med. *125* (1955), 401—408.
247. Schmidt, H. W., Über Anordnung und Hämodynamik der arterio-arteriellen Anastomosen in der Pia mater. Z. Ges. Exp. Med. *125* (1955), 229—235.
248. Schmidt, H. W., Experimentelle Untersuchungen zur Frage der Gefäß-spasmen in den extrakraniellen Carotis-Anteilen bei der cerebralen Angiographie. Dtsch. Z. Nervenheilk. *174* (1956), 173—176.
249. Schmidt, H. W., Tierexperimentelle Untersuchungen zur Frage der Gefäß-spasmen bei Hirnembolie. Dtsch. Z. Nervenheilk. *174* (1956), 499—504.
250. Schmidt, H. W., Reaktion der Piagefäße auf Röntgenkontrastmittel bei geschädigtem Gehirnkreislauf. Dtsch. Z. Nervenheilk. *174* (1956), 167—172.
251. Schutta, H. S., Kassel, N. F., Langfitt, T. W., Brain swelling produced by injury and aggravated by arterial hypertension. Brain *91* (1968), 281—294.
252. Schwab, M., Das Säure-Basen-Gleichgewicht im arteriellen Blut und Liquor cerebrospinalis bei chronischer Niereninsuffizienz. Klin. Wschr. *41* (1962), 765—772.
253. Sercombe, R., Aubineau, P., Edvinsson, L., Mamo, H., Owman, Ch., Pinard, E., Seylaz, J., Neurogenic influence on local cerebral blood flow: effect of catecholamines or sympathetic stimulation as correlated with the sympathetic innervation. Neurol. *25* (1975), 954—963.
254. Severinghaus, J. W., Lassen, N. A., Step hypocapnia to separate arterial from tissue pCO_2 in the regulation of cerebral blood flow. Circ. Res. *20* (1967), 272—278.
255. Severinghaus, J. W., Coupling mechanisms flow to function and metabolism in brain, a general discussion. In: Brain work, pp. 503—517. Eds.: Ingvar, D. H., Lassen, N. A. Copenhagen: Munksgaard. 1975.
256. Severs, W. B., Daniels-Severs, A. E., Effects of angiotensin on the central nervous system. Pharmacol. Rev. *23* (1973), 415—449.
257. Shapiro, H. M., Stromberg, D. D., Lee, D. R., Wiederhelm, C. A., Dynamic pressures in the pial arterial microcirculation. Amer. J. Physiol. *221* (1971), 279—283.
258. Shelden, C. H., Pudenz, R. H., Restonska, J. S., Craig, W. M., The lucite calvarium—a method for direct observation of the brain. I. The surgical and lucite processing techniques. J. Neurosurg. *1* (1944), 67—69.
259. Silvertsson, R., Hemodynamic importance of structural vascular changes in essential hypertension. Acta Physiol. Scand. Suppl. *343* (1970), 1—56.
260. Skinhøj, E., Strandgaard, S., Pathogenesis of hypertensive encephalopathy. Lancet *1* (1973), 461—462.
261. Sohler, T. P., Lothrop, G. N., Forbes, H. S., The pial circulation of normal, non-anaesthetized animals. II. The effect of drugs, alcohol and CO_2. J. Pharmac. exp. Ther. *71* (1941), 331—335.
262. Sokoloff, L., The action of drugs on the cerebral circulation. Pharmacol. Rev. *11* (1959), 1—58.
263. Sondaki, S., Joó, F., Maurer, M., The permeability state of the blood brain barrier in relation with the plasma-renin activity in early stage of experimental renal hypertension. Brit. J. exp. Path. *51* (1970), 448—452.

264. Steinwall, O., Klatzo, I., Selective vulnerability of the blood brain barrier in chemically induced lesions. J. Neuropath. exp. Neurol. 25 (1966), 542—559.

265. Stone, H. L., Raichle, M. E., Hernandez, M., The effect of sympathetic denervation on cerebral CO_2 sensitivity. Stroke 5 (1974), 13—18.

266. Strandgaard, S., Olesen, J., Skinhøj, E., Lassen, N. A., Autoregulation of brain circulation in severe arterial hypertension. Brit. Med. J. 1 (1973), 507—510.

267. Strandgaard, S., MacKenzie, E. T., Sengupta, D., Rowan, J. O., Lassen, N. A., Harper, A. M., Upper limit of autoregulation of cerebral blood flow in the baboon. Circ. Res. 24 (1974), 435—440.

268. Strandgaard, S., MacKenzie, E. T., Jones, J. V., Harper, A. M., Studies on cerebral blood flow following "breakthrough" of autoregulation. In: Blood flow and metabolism in the brain, pp. 5.15.—5.16. Eds.: Harper, A. M., Jennett, W. B., Miller, J. D., Rowan, J. O. Edinburgh: Churchill Livingstone. 1975.

269. Strandgaard, S., Jones, J. V., MacKenzie, E. T., Harper, A. M., Upper limit of cerebral blood flow autoregulation in experimental renovascular hypertension in the baboon. Circ. Res. 37 (1975), 164—167.

270. Strandgaard, S., MacKenzie, E. T., Jones, J. V., Harper, A. M., Studies on the cerebral circulation of the baboon in acutely induced hypertension. Stroke 7 (1976), 287—290.

271. Strandgaard, S., Jones, J. V., MacKenzie, E. T., Graham, D. I., Farrar, J. K., The sausage string pattern in the pial vessels in acute, angiotensin-induced hypertension—vasospasm or vasodilatation? Acta Med. Scand. Suppl. (1976), 9—12.

272. Stromberg, D. D., Fox, J. R., Pressures in the pial arterial microcirculation of the cat during changes in systemic arterial blood pressure. Circ. Res. 31 (1972), 229—239.

273. Suzuki, T., Response of pial microcirculation to changes in arterial carbon dioxide tension and to reduction in systemic blood pressure. J. of Jap. Coll. Angiol. 15 (1975), 171—178.

274. Suzuki, T., Tominaga, S., Strandgaard, S., Nakamura, T., Fluorescein cineangiography of the pial microcirculation in the rat in acute angiotensininduced hypertension. In: Blood flow and metabolism in the brain, pp. 5.8.—5.9. Eds.: Harper, A. M., Jennett, W. B., Miller, J. D., Rowan, J. O., Edinburgh: Churchill Livingstone. 1975.

275. Symon, L., Held, K., Dorsch, N. W. C., On the myogenic nature of the autoregulatory mechanism in the cerebral circulation. Europ. Neurol. 6 (1971/72), 11—18.

276. Teichmann, K., Beobachtungen über Stoffaustausch im Kapillargebiet mit Hilfe der intravitalen Fluoreszenzmikroskopie. Z. d. ges. exp. Med. 110 (1942), 723—745.

277. Thurel, R., Cerebromeningeal edema due to arterial hypertension. Arch. Neurol. Psychiat. 69 (1953), 140.

278. Traystman, R. J., Rapela, C. E., Effect of sympathetic nerve stimulation on cerebral and cephalic blood flow in dogs. Circ. Res. 36 (1975), 620—630.

279. Villaret, M., Les répercussions vasculaires tardives de l'embolie cérébrale (en pathologie expérimentale). La Presse Médicale 47 (1939), 267—271.

280. Vonwiller, P., Neue Wege der Gewebelehre des Menschen und der Tiere. Zbl. Allg. Path. und Path. Anat. 33 (1923), 12—38.

281. Wahl, M., Deetjen, P., Thurau, K., Ingvar, D. H., Lassen, N. A., Micropuncture evaluation of the importance of perivascular pH for the arteriolar diameter on the brain surface. Pflügers Archiv *316* (1970), 152—163.
282. Wahl, M., Kuschinsky, W., Bosse, O., Oleson, J., Lassen, N. A., Ingvar, D. H., Michaelis, J., Thurau, K., Effect of 1-norepinephrine on the diameter of pial arterioles and arteries in the rat. Circ. Res. *31* (1972), 248—256.
283. Wahl, M., Kuschinsky, W., Bosse, O., Thurau, K., Dependency of pial arterial and arteriolar diameter on perivascular osmolarity in the cat. Circ. Res. *32* (1973), 162—169.
284. Walter, G. F., Auer, L., Auböck, W., Brain edema in acute arterial hypertension. III. Electron microscopic results. In prep.
285. Waltz, A. G., Yamaguchi, T., Regli, F., Regulatory responses of cerebral vasculature after sympathetic denervation. Amer. J. Physiol. *221* (1971), 298—302.
286. Weinstein, J. D., Langfitt, T. W., Kassel, N. F., Vasopressor response to increased intracranial pressure. Neurol. *14* (1964), 1118—1131.
287. Westergaard, E., Van Deurs, B., Brøndsted, H. E., Increased vesicular transfer of horseradish peroxidase across cerebral endothelium, evoked by acute hypertension. Acta Neuropath. *37* (1977), 141—152.
288. Westergaard, E., Transport of protein tracers across cerebral arterioles under normal condition. In: Pathology of cerebral microcirculation, pp. 218—227. Ed.: Cervos-Navarro, J. Berlin: Walter de Gruyter. 1974.
289. Wolff, H. G., The cerebral circulation. XI a. The action of acetylcholine. Arch. Neurol. Psychiat. *22* (1929), 686—699.
290. Wolff, H. G., The cerebral circulation. XII. Arch. Neurol. Psychiat. *23* (1930), 1097—1120.
291. Yoshida, K., Meyer, J. S., Sakamoto, K., Handa, J., Autoregulation of cerebral blood flow—electromagnetic flow measurements during acute hypertension in the monkey. Circ. Res. *19* (1966), 726—738.
292. Zimmermann, B. G., Drug action on peripheral vascular system. Ann. Rev. Pharm. *2* (1972), 125—140.
293. Zweifach, B. W., General principles governing the behaviour of the microcirculation. Amer. J. Med. *23* (1957), 684—696.
294. Zweifach, B. W., Direct observation of the mesenteric circulation in experimental animals Anat. Rec. *120* (1954), 277—291.